Simulation in Cardiovascular Critical Care Medicine

Ronald A. Bronicki • Sebastian C. Tume
Daniel Burkhoff • Daniel J. Penny
Editors

Simulation in Cardiovascular Critical Care Medicine

Integration of Pathophysiology, Monitoring, and Therapy

Springer

Editors
Ronald A. Bronicki
Department of Pediatrics
Texas Children's Hospital Baylor College of Medicine, Suite E1420
Houston, TX, USA

Sebastian C. Tume
Department of Pediatrics
Texas Children's Hospital Baylor College of Medicine
Houston, TX, USA

Daniel Burkhoff
Cardiovascular Research Foundation
New York, NY, USA

Daniel J. Penny
Baylor College of Medicine
Texas Children's Hospital
Houston, TX, USA

ISBN 978-3-031-63556-4 ISBN 978-3-031-63557-1 (eBook)
https://doi.org/10.1007/978-3-031-63557-1

This Springer imprint is published by the registered company Springer Nature Switzerland AG
The registered company address is: Gewerbestrasse 11, 6330 Cham, Switzerland

To my parents, Meyer and Shoshana, thank you for demonstrating the importance of dedication and perseverance, and to my wife, Katie, and children, Abigail and Jacob, thank you for all of your love and support.

Ronald A. Bronicki

To my cherished patients and their families whose resilience and trust fuels my commitment to improve the care I give every day. Thank you for allowing me to join you on your journey as we navigate challenges with empathy and hope.

Daniel J. Penny

Contents

Contributors

Alex Alali University of Pennsylvania Perelman School of Medicine, Children's Hospital of Philadelphia, Philadelphia, PA, USA

Nirica Borges Baylor College of Medicine, Texas Children's Hospital, Houston, TX, USA

Ronald A. Bronicki Baylor College of Medicine, Texas Children's Hospital, Houston, TX, USA

Daniel Burkhoff Cardiovascular Research Foundation, New York, NY, USA

John M. Costello Medical University of South Carolina, Shawn Jenkins Children's Hospital, Charleston, SC, USA

Cameron Dezfulian Baylor College of Medicine, Texas Children's Hospital, Houston, TX, USA

Saul Flores Baylor College of Medicine, Texas Children's Hospital, Houston, TX, USA

Hernando Gomez University of Pittsburgh School of Medicine, Pittsburgh, PA, USA

Kyle D. Hope Baylor College of Medicine, Texas Children's Hospital, Houston, TX, USA

Javier J. Lasa University of Texas Southwestern Medical School, Children's Medical Center of Dallas, Dallas, TX, USA

Rohit S. Loomba Chicago Medical School/Rosalind Franklin University of Medicine, Advocate Children's Hospital, Chicago, IL, USA

Daniel J. Penny Baylor College of Medicine, Texas Children's Hospital, Houston, TX, USA

Joseph Philip University of Florida College of Medicine, University of Florida Health Shands Hospital, Gainesville, FL, USA

Michael R. Pinsky University of Pittsburgh School of Medicine, Pittsburgh, PA, USA

Khayri Shalhoub Baylor College of Medicine, Texas Children's Hospital, Houston, TX, USA

Kriti Puri Baylor College of Medicine, Texas Children's Hospital, Houston, TX, USA

Jordan Schneider Central Michigan University College of Medicine, Children's Hospital of Michigan, Detroit, MI, USA

Lara S. Shekerdemian Baylor College of Medicine, Texas Children's Hospital, Houston, TX, USA

Sebastian C. Tume Baylor College of Medicine, Texas Children's Hospital, Houston, TX, USA

Abbreviations

AR	aortic regurgitation
AS	aortic stenosis
AVP	arginine vasopressin
BP	blood pressure
CO	cardiac output
CPP	coronary perfusion pressure
DB	dobutamine
DO_2	oxygen delivery
EDV	end diastolic volume
ESV	end systolic volume
EDPVR	end diastolic pressure volume relationship
ESPVR	end systolic pressure volume relationship
Ees	ventricular elastance
Ea	arterial elastance
EF	ejection fraction
HF	heart failure
HR	heart rate
LV	left ventricle
LVAD	left ventricular assist device
mPAP	mean pulmonary artery pressure
MR	mitral regurgitation
NE	norepinephrine
NTP	nitroprusside
PA	pulmonary artery
PAOP	pulmonary artery occlusion pressure
PE	potential energy
PHTN	pulmonary hypertension
PVL	pressure volume loop
PVA	pressure volume area
Pes	pressure end systolic
RF	regurgitant fraction

RV	right ventricle
SBV	stressed blood volume
SV	stroke volume
SVR	systemic vascular resistance
SW	stroke work
VA ECMO	venoarterial extracorporeal membrane oxygenation
Vo	volume axis intercept
VO_2	oxygen consumption
WU	Wood unit

Chapter 1
Introduction

Ronald A. Bronicki and Daniel J. Penny

The overarching goal in medicine is to do the right thing for the right patient at the right time. There are several challenges to accomplishing this task. The presentation and evolution of disease varies from one patient to the next, necessitating a tailored approach and avoidance of a "one-size-fits-all" approach to patient care [1–6]. Clinical practice guidelines and protocols should not be prescriptive, and clinicians should adhere to or diverge from them as needed. This approach is predicated on establishing the underlying pathophysiology and tailoring therapies accordingly. A thorough understanding and application of physiology and pathophysiology and advanced monitoring is essential to accomplishing this goal. Nowhere is this more evident than in the practice of critical care medicine [1–3].

Cardiovascular physiology and pathophysiology play a prominent role in many disease processes, either precipitating or contributing to the evolution of disease [7, 8]. Establishing the baseline hemodynamic phenotype is essential to selecting optimal therapies. However, there are obstacles to accomplishing this task. First, clinical examination and standard hemodynamic monitoring, in both adults and children, do not reliably predict quantitative measures of cardiovascular function [9–17]. This has been demonstrated in those presenting with acute severe illness as well as those evaluated during the chronic convalescent state and in those with or without primary cardiovascular disease [9–17]. These inaccuracies have been shown to occur irrespective of the level and nature of training of the physicians providing the assessment [9, 16].

For reasons such as these, multi-societal consensus-driven guidelines recommend the use of advanced hemodynamic monitoring in the management of critically ill children and adults to establish the hemodynamic phenotype and guide therapy [3, 18, 19]. The use of advanced hemodynamic monitoring however has

R. A. Bronicki (✉) · D. J. Penny
Baylor College of Medicine, Texas Children's Hospital, Houston, TX, USA
e-mail: rxbronic@texaschildrens.org; djpenny@texaschildrens.org

R. A. Bronicki et al. (eds.), *Simulation in Cardiovascular Critical Care Medicine*, https://doi.org/10.1007/978-3-031-63557-1_1

come under considerable scrutiny due to the inherent risk of invasive monitoring and the lack of evidence demonstrating improved outcomes [20–22], and studies have shown that there are shortcomings in clinical reasoning [23–25], deficiencies in knowledge [25–27], and a lack of proficiency in interpretating advanced hemodynamic monitoring [28–33].

A further challenge for the clinician is the dynamic nature of disease processes, and the impact of therapeutic interventions on cardiovascular function, necessitating an ongoing assessment of the pathophysiologic profile. Organ interactions amplify the complexity of critical illness, with cardio-renal and cardio-pulmonary interactions contributing importantly to the pathophysiology and the selection of optimal therapies, for example.

For these reasons, we will utilize the ventricular pressure-volume diagram and time-varying elastance framework to provide a foundation for understanding: cardiovascular physiology and pathophysiology; the interpretation and limitations of standard and advanced hemodynamic monitoring devices; the physiologic basis and hemodynamic effects of therapeutic interventions; and the physiologic underpinnings and clinical relevance of heart lung interactions in the care of critically ill patients. We will build on this foundation by utilizing a cardiovascular simulator to illustrate the application of these important principles in the care of patients with critical cardiac disease.

Simulation is ideally suited to enhance our understanding of the complexities of the cardiovascular system, which is a closed-loop hydrodynamic system with complex heart and vascular interactions. In this review, we use the Harvi cardiovascular simulator (PVLoops, LLC) in which each chamber of the heart is represented by a time-varying elastance, and the systemic and pulmonary vasculature are represented by the three elements of the modified Windkessel model [34–36]. The simulator generates ventricular pressure-volume loops from each of the four chambers, time-dependent tracings of pressures, flows and volumes, and the hemodynamic parameters derived from these signals. The hemodynamic values are provided for illustrative purposes. The changes in magnitude of these parameters may vary depending on the host response to the therapy.

The simulator has been summarized and validated as described in previous publications [37–39]. The simulator illustrates complex physiological principles, which may be used to enhance our understanding of diseases processes; predict the impact of therapeutic interventions; and demonstrate how even the most complex pathophysiological abnormalities alter clinical parameters used by the clinician at the bedside [40–49].

References

1. Tobin MJ. Why physiology is critical to the practice of medicine. A 40-year personal perspective. Clin Chest Med. 2019;40:243–57.

2. Gattinoni L, Carlesso E, Santini A. Physiology versus evidence-based guidance for critical care practice. Crit Care. 2015;19:57.
3. Tonelli MR, Curtis JR, Guntupalli KK, et al. An official multi-society statement: the role of clinical research results in the practice of critical care medicine. Am J Respir Crit Care Med. 2012;185:1117–24.
4. Guarracino F, Bertini P, Pinsky MR. Heterogeneity of cardiovascular response to standardized sepsis resuscitation. Crit Care. 2020;24:99.
5. Ceneviva G, Paschall A, Maffei F, et al. Hemodynamic support in fluid-refractory pediatric septic shock. Pediatrics. 1998;102:e19.
6. De Backer D, Vieillard-Baron A. Clinical examination: a trigger but not a substitute for hemodynamic evaluation. Intensive Care Med. 2019;45:269–71.
7. Meert KL, Banks R, Holubkov R, et al. Morbidity and mortality in critically ill children. II. A qualitative patient-level analysis of pathophysiologies and potential therapeutic solutions. Crit Care Med. 2020;48:799–807.
8. Morrow DA, Fang JC, Fintel DJ, et al. Evolution of critical care cardiology: transformation of the cardiovascular intensive care unit and the emerging need for new medical staffing and training models: a scientific statement from the American Heart Association. Circulation. 2012;126:1408–28.
9. Tibby SM, Hatherill M, Marsh MJ, et al. Clinicians' abilities to estimate cardiac index in ventilated children and infants. Arch Dis Child. 1997;77:516–8.
10. Connors JAF, McCaffree DR, Gray BA. Evaluation of right-heart catheterization in the critically ill patient without acute myocardial infarction. N Engl J Med. 1983;308:263–7.
11. Stevenson LW, Perloff JK. The limited reliability of physical signs for estimating hemodynamics in chronic heart failure. JAMA. 1989;261:884–8.
12. Eagle KA, Quertermous T, Singer DE, et al. Left ventricular ejection fraction. Physician estimates compared with gated blood pool scan measurements. Arch Intern Med. 1988;148:882–5.
13. Marantz PR, Tobin JN, Wassertheil-Smoller S, Steingart RM, et al. The relationship between left ventricular systolic function and congestive heart failure diagnosed by clinical criteria. Circulation. 1988;77:607–12.
14. Mimoz O, Rauss A, Rekik N, et al. Pulmonary artery catheterization in critically ill patients: a prospective analysis of outcome changes associated with catheter-prompted changes in therapy. Crit Care Med. 1994;22:573–9.
15. Eisenberg PR, Jaffe AS, Schuster DP. Clinical evaluation compared to pulmonary artery catheterization in the hemodynamic assessment of critically ill patients. Crit Care Med. 1984;12:549–53.
16. Narang N, Chung B, Nguyen A, et al. Discordance between clinical assessment and invasive hemodynamics in patients with advanced heart failure. J Card Fail. 2020;26:128–35.
17. Connors JRAF, Speroff T, Dawson NV, et al. The effectiveness of right heart catheterization in the initial care of critically ill patients. JAMA. 1996;276:889–97.
18. Weiss SL, Peters MJ, Alhazzani W, et al. Surviving sepsis campaign international guidelines for the management of septic shock and sepsis-associated organ dysfunction in children. Pediatr Crit Care Med. 2020;21:e52–e106.
19. Cecconi M, De Backer D, Antonelli M, et al. Consensus on circulatory shock and hemodynamic monitoring. Task force of the European Society of Intensive Care Medicine. Intensive Care Med. 2014;40:1795–815.
20. The ESCAPE Investigators and ESCAPE Study Coordinators. Evaluation study of congestive heart failure and pulmonary artery catheterization effectiveness. JAMA. 2005;294:1625–33.
21. Harvey S, Harrison DA, Singer M, et al. Assessment of the clinical effectiveness of pulmonary artery catheters in management of patients in intensive care (PAC-Man): a randomized controlled trial. Lancet. 2005;366:472–7.
22. Chatterjee K. The Swan-Ganz catheters: past, present, and future. A viewpoint. Circulation. 2009;119:147–52.

23. Simpkin AL, Schwartzstein RM. Tolerating uncertainty—the next medical revolution? N Engl J Med. 2016;375:1713–5.
24. Croskerry P. From mindless to mindful practice—cognitive bias and clinical decision making. N Engl J Med. 2013;368:2445–8.
25. Norman GR, Monteiro SD, Sherbino J, et al. The causes of errors in clinical reasoning: cognitive biases, knowledge deficits, and dual process thinking. Acad Med. 2017;92:23–30.
26. Royce CS, Hayes MM, Schwartzstein RM. Teaching critical thinking: a case for instruction in cognitive biases to reduce diagnostic errors and improve patient safety. Acad Med. 2019;94:187–94.
27. Morris AH. Human cognitive limitations. Broad, consistent, clinical application of physiological principles will require decision support. Ann Am Thorac Soc. 2018;15:S53–6.
28. Gnaegi A, Feihl F, Perret C. Intensive care physicians' insufficient of right heart catheterization at the bedside: time to act? Crit Care Med. 1997;25:213–20.
29. Iberti TJ, Fischer EP, Leibowitz AB, et al. A multicenter study of physicians' knowledge of the pulmonary artery catheter. JAMA. 1990;264:2928–32.
30. Boerma EC, Bootsma IT. Physician factors in utilizing haemodynamic data in patient care. Curr Opin Crit Care. 2019;25:292–7.
31. Squara P, Bennett D, Perret C. Pulmonary artery catheter. Does the problem lie in the users? Chest. 2002;121:2009–15.
32. Perel A, Saugel B, Teboul JL, et al. The effects of advanced monitoring on hemodynamic management in critically ill patients: a pre and post questionnaire study. J Clin Monit Comput. 2016;30:511–8.
33. Saugel B, Malbrain M, Perel A. Hemodynamic monitoring in the era of evidence-based medicine. Crit Care. 2016;20:401.
34. Suga H, Sagawa K. Instantaneous pressure-volume relationships and their ratio in the excised, supported canine left ventricle. Circ Res. 1974;35:117–26.
35. Sunagawa K, Maughan L, Burkhoff D, et al. Left ventricular interaction with arterial load studied in isolated canine ventricle. Am J Phys. 1983;245:H773–80.
36. Guyton AC. Determination of cardiac output by equating venous return curves with cardiac response curves. Physiol Rev. 1955;35:123–9.
37. Burkhoff D, Tyberg JV. Why does pulmonary venous pressure rise after onset of LV dysfunction: a theoretical analysis. Am J Phys. 1993;265:H1819–28.
38. Doshi D, Burkhoff D. Cardiovascular simulation of heart failure pathophysiology and therapeutics. J Card Fail. 2016;22:303–11.
39. Burkhoff D, Mirsky I, Suga H. Assessment of systolic and diastolic ventricular properties via pressure-volume analysis: a guide for clinical, translational, and basic researchers. Am J Physiol Heart Circ Physiol. 2005;289:H501–12.
40. Tanaka K, Oshita S, Kitahata H, et al. Effects of nicardipine on ventriculo-arterial coupling in humans. Br J Anaesth. 1998;81:180–5.
41. Yamamoto K, Kodama K, Masuyama T, et al. Adverse effects of epinephrine in patients with advanced left ventricular dysfunction: analysis of ventriculo-arterial coupling. Int J Cardiol. 1992;32:143–55.
42. Chantler PD, Lakatta EG, Najjar SS. Arterial-ventricular coupling: mechanistic insights into cardiovascular performance at rest and during exercise. J Appl Physiol. 2008;105:1342–51.
43. Bastos MB, Burkhoff D, Maly J, et al. Invasive left ventricle pressure-volume analysis: overview and practical clinical implications. Eur Heart J. 2020;41:1286–97.
44. Burkhoff D. Pressure-volume loops in clinical research. J Am Coll Cardiol. 2013;62:1173–6.
45. Pinsky MR, Guarracino F. How to assess ventriculoarterial coupling in sepsis. Curr Opin Crit Care. 2020;26:313–8.
46. Guarracino F, Bertini P, Pinsky MR. Cardiovascular determinants of resuscitation from sepsis and septic shock. Crit Care. 2019;23:118.
47. Guarracino F, Ferro B, Morelli A, et al. Ventriculoarterial decoupling in human septic shock. Crit Care. 2014;18:R80.

48. Ky B, French B, May KA, et al. Ventricular-arterial coupling, remodeling, and prognosis in chronic heart failure. J Am Coll Cardiol. 2013;62:1165–72.
49. Nishio R, Sasayama S, Matsumori A. Left ventricular pressure-volume relationship in a murine model of congestive heart failure due to acute viral myocarditis. J Am Coll Cardiol. 2002;40:1506–14.

Chapter 2
Ventricular Pressure-Volume Relationship and Time-Varying Elastance Model

Ronald A. Bronicki, Daniel J. Penny, and Daniel Burkhoff

Introduction

The utility of the ventricular pressure-volume loop (PVL) and the ventricular pressure-volume relationship to characterize and quantify the mechanical properties of the left ventricle (LV) was demonstrated by Otto Frank in 1895 [1]. Using isolated frog hearts, Frank illustrated the changes in ventricular pressure and volume throughout the cardiac cycle and that the minimum and maximum pressures within the ventricle (the end-diastolic and end-systolic pressure-volume relationships, respectively) were highly dependent on the extent of filling prior to the onset of contraction (preload) and the pressure against which the ventricle ejected (afterload).

Suga and colleagues extended the work of Frank by analyzing the time-varying ratio of instantaneous pressure to instantaneous volume in the canine LV and introduced a load-independent index of LV contractility in 1969 [2]. Subsequent work by Suga, Sunagawa, and others demonstrated that this time-varying elastance model was also valid for describing right ventricular (RV) and atrial properties; established a framework for analyzing the interaction between a ventricle and its arterial system by also characterizing the arterial load in terms of a pressure-volume relationship [3]; and demonstrated the correlation between total ventricular mechanical work and myocardial oxygen consumption (VO_2) [4]. These principles provide the basis for our discussion of cardiovascular physiology and pathophysiology and for predicting the impact of therapies.

R. A. Bronicki (✉) · D. J. Penny
Baylor College of Medicine, Texas Children's Hospital, Houston, TX, USA
e-mail: rxbronic@texaschildrens.org; djpenny@texaschildrens.org

D. Burkhoff
Cardiovascular Research Foundation, New York, NY, USA
e-mail: dburkhoff@crf.org

R. A. Bronicki et al. (eds.), *Simulation in Cardiovascular Critical Care Medicine*, https://doi.org/10.1007/978-3-031-63557-1_2

Ventricular Pressure-Volume Diagram

With each cardiac cycle, chamber muscle contracts and stiffens, reaching maximal stiffness at end systole, and then relaxes, reaching minimal stiffness at end diastole. The mechanical properties of the heart chambers are thus time-varying, varying in a cyclic manner. We will examine the time-varying mechanical properties of the ventricle throughout the cardiac cycle using the pressure-volume diagram and during extremes in stiffness by examining the end-systolic and end-diastolic pressure-volume relationships (ESPVR, EDPVR).

The PVL begins with contraction and the isovolumic phase of the cardiac cycle. Ventricular ejection begins once ventricular pressure rises above aortic pressure (Fig. 2.1). Peak LV pressure is similar to peak aortic pressure or systolic blood pressure, which is followed by the end-systolic pressure (Pes). This is followed by the isovolumic relaxation phase and then ventricular filling phase of the cardiac cycle once atrial pressure exceeds ventricular pressure. The difference between end-systolic volume (ESV) and end-diastolic volume (EDV) is stroke volume (SV).

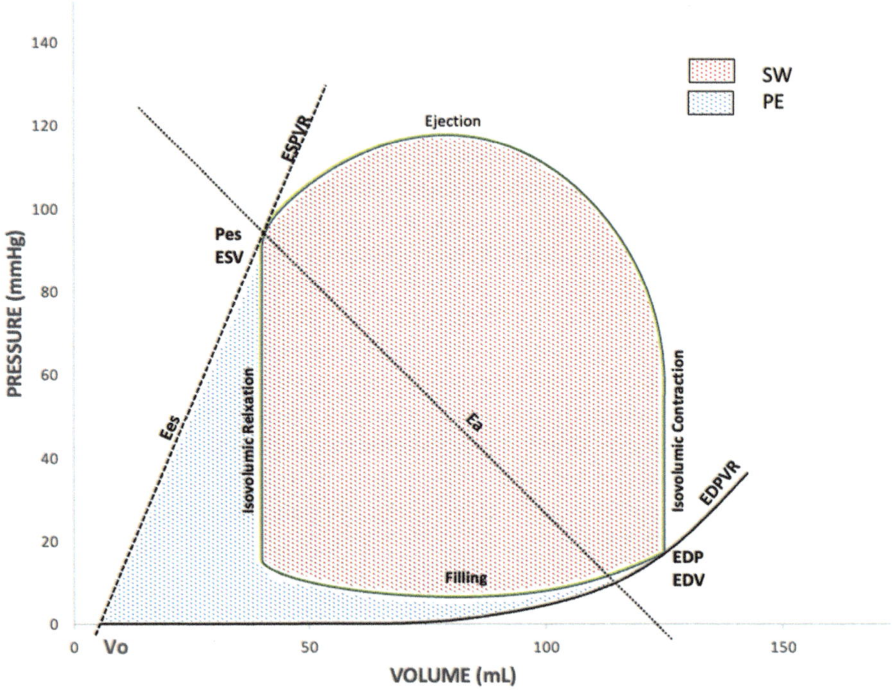

Fig. 2.1 *Ventricular pressure volume loop.* The cardiac cycle begins with the isovolumic phase of contraction. Ventricular ejection begins once ventricular pressure rises above aortic pressure. Peak LV pressure is similar to peak aortic pressure or systolic BP, which is followed by Pes. This is followed by the isovolumic relaxation phase of diastole and then ventricular filling phase of the cardiac cycle once atrial pressure exceeds ventricular pressure. The difference between ESV and EDV is SV

The End-Diastolic Pressure-Volume Relationship

The EDPRV is established by altering ventricular loading conditions and generating a series of PVLs and connecting the end-diastolic pressure-volume points of each loop. The EDPVR is curvilinear in nature and is indicative of ventricular passive viscoelastic properties or stiffness at the point of complete myofilament inactivation (Fig. 2.1). Chamber stiffness, or its reciprocal, chamber compliance, relates changes in ventricular volume in response to changes in the diastolic transmural pressure. A shift upward and leftward in the EDPVR is indicative of an increase in stiffness; a shift downward and rightward is indicative of a decrease in ventricular stiffness (Fig. 2.2) [5]. For a given EDPVR, as volume increases, the pressure begins to rise, and with large volume, the pressure increases disproportionately. That is to say that *operating chamber stiffness* increases at higher volumes (volume-dependent changes in chamber stiffness) [6]. The maximal volume along the EDPRV at which the pressure remains zero is referred to as the unstressed volume, Vo (Fig. 2.1) [5].

The determinants of ventricular stiffness are ventricular or chamber geometry (ventricular muscle mass or wall thickness to EDV ratio) and the material properties

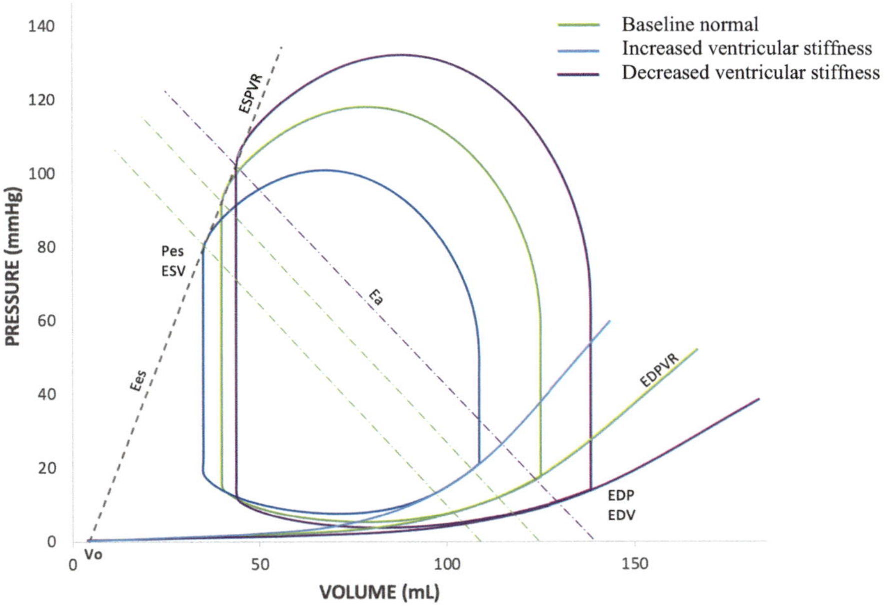

Fig. 2.2 *Altered ventricular stiffness.* LV PVLs illustrating isolated changes in ventricular stiffness. An increase in ventricular stiffness, or decrease in compliance, is indicated by a shift of the EDPVR up and to the left. When ventricular stiffness is elevated, a higher ventricular diastolic transmural pressure is required to generate the same EDV as in a ventricle with normal stiffness. Also, an increase in ventricular stiffness does not necessarily equate with an elevated EDP. The EDP is the result of ventricular stiffness and the extent of ventricular filling (EDV)

of the myocardium [5–10]. Changes in chamber geometry may result from physiologic (e.g., exercise-induced) or pathologic processes (pressure and/or volume overload) and may be acute (e.g., following repair of mitral regurgitation) or chronic in nature (e.g., aortic stenosis induced ventricular hypertrophy). These processes and their clinical impact will be discussed in detail with specific lesions.

Myocardial stiffness refers to the intrinsic properties of the myocardium and is reflected in the myocardial stress-strain relationship, the resistance of the myocardium to stretch when subjected to stress. This relationship defines myocardial stiffness irrespective of the effects it may have upon ventricular or chamber stiffness. Alterations in myocardial properties result from changes in the cardiomyocyte and/or extracellular matrix and may occur acutely (e.g., inflammation and edema resulting from ischemia-reperfusion injury) or be the result of a chronic process (e.g., alterations in collagen metabolism) [5–10].

Other factors external to the heart may alter the effective compliance of the entire heart. As intrathoracic pressure increases, for example, the surrounding pressure of the heart increases, and as a result the diastolic transmural pressure and the effective compliance for each chamber decrease. The extent to which this occurs depends on the magnitude of change in airway pressure and the extent to which this change in airway pressure is transmitted to the cardiac fossa (see Chap. 5 on heart lung interactions). Similarly, pericardial disease may alter the effective compliance of the heart, depending in part on the rate of development and the magnitude of the lesion. Another important factor that affects the rate and extent of ventricular filling and thus ventricular diastolic volume and pressure is the process of myocardial relaxation, which is discussed in detail in Chap. 3 on diastolic function.

End-Systolic Pressure-Volume Relationship

The ESPVR reflects the stiffness of the ventricular chamber at the point of maximum myofilament activation. It is examined by altering ventricular loading conditions and generating a series of PVLs and connecting the end-systolic pressure-volume points of each loop (Fig. 2.1). The relationship between ventricular pressure and volume at end systole (the ESPVR) was demonstrated to be reasonably linear over the working pressure-volume range of the heart by Suga and colleagues who first used it as a load-independent index of contractility [2].

The ESPVR is quantified by a slope referred to as end-systolic elastance (Ees), where Es (mmHg/ml) = Pes/ESV − Vo, and Vo is the volume axis intercept of the ESPVR, obtained from the linear extrapolation of the ESPVR. The positive value for Vo of the ESPVR indicates that a finite amount of ventricular volume is needed

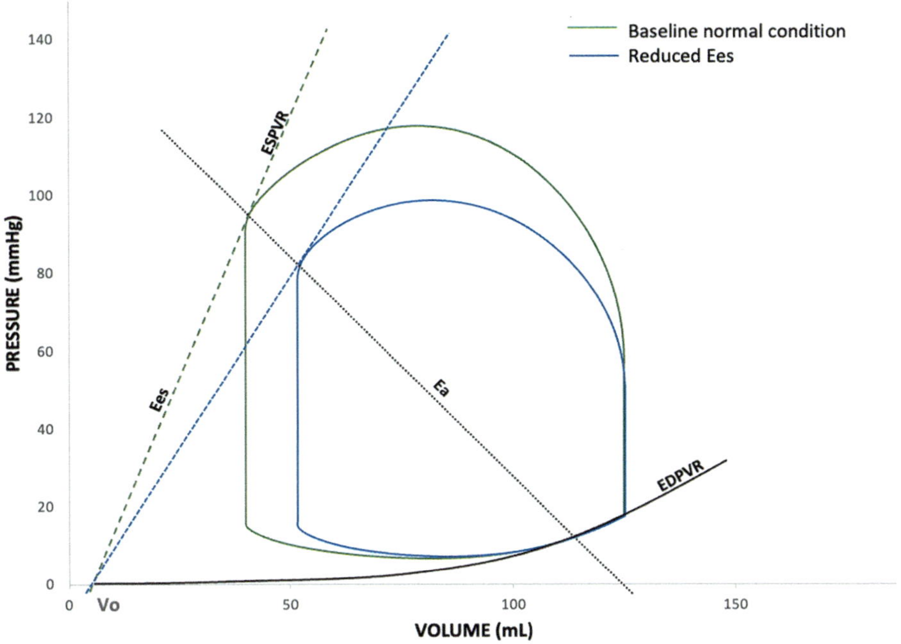

Fig. 2.3 *Alterations in ventricular contractility.* Ventricular PVLs illustrating the impact of an isolated decrease in ventricular Ees. The arterial load Ea is unchanged, Ees has decreased, thus Ea/Ees has increased. As a result, the EF and SV have decreased. Pes has decreased because Ea is unchanged and Ees has decreased. Ventricular afterload (systolic BP) and the PVA have also decreased

before it can generate pressure. With acute alterations in contractility, the slope of Ees changes accordingly with little change in Vo [5]. Figure 2.3 illustrates the effects of isolated changes in LV Ees on SV and Pes.

With extreme changes in contractility and in hearts that have undergone significant remodeling, several factors must be considered when interpreting Ees as an index of contractility [5]. With significant remodeling and enlargement, Vo may increase. Second, the ESPVR may become nonlinear, in which case the extrapolated value of Vo may differ from actual. This occurs with marked reductions in contractility and in hearts that have undergone significant remodeling and ventricular enlargement [5]. For these reasons, the ESPVR is well approximated by a straight line over a limited working range of pressures and volumes; however, extrapolation to the low-pressure range may not be accurate [5]. Thus, when quantifying changes in LV contractility, changes in both Ees and Vo must be considered [5]. There are several combinations of changes in Ees and Vo that are consistent with an increase in contractility. Ees increases, with little change in Vo; Ees remains unchanged, however Vo decreases; Ees and Vo both decrease; and Ees and Vo both increase. In each case, within the specified working range of pressure and volume, an increase in contractility is reflected in an increase in end-systolic pressure generation at a common volume.

Arterial Elastance

Sunagawa and colleagues followed by developing a theoretical framework and graphical representation to explain how the ventricle interacts with its arterial system to determine SV and pressure (Pes) [3]. This approach requires the arterial load to also be represented in the pressure-volume plane. Like the ventricle, the arterial system may also be viewed as an elastic chamber (arterial elastance, Ea, in mmHg/ml) that undergoes cyclic changes in pressure relative to volume, with the distribution of volume (SV) between the two chambers determined by the relative elastance (Ea/Ees) [3, 11]. However, because the major determinant of arterial elastance is not the physical compliance of the arterial system but resistance, it is referred to as "effective elastance" [11].

Based on the three-element Windkessel model of the vasculature, Sunagawa and colleagues derived Ea to represent the arterial load, incorporating the steady, non-pulsatile (peripheral resistance), and pulsatile components (compliance and characteristic impedance).

This approach relies on simplifying assumptions applied to a basic principle of hemodynamics: Total peripheral resistance (TPR) = mean arterial pressure (MAP)—CVP/CO or MAP—CVP/SV X HR. If the CVP is negligible relative to the MAP and the MAP can be approximated by Pes, the equation may be rearranged to: TPR X HR $\cong$ Pes/SV = Ea. On the PVL, Ea is represented graphically by the negative slope connecting the EDV at zero pressure to the end-systolic pressure-volume coordinate [3, 11, 12] (Fig. 2.1). A third assumption is that the volume at end ejection is equivalent to the volume at end systole, which is the point on the PVL that intersects with the ESPVR. These assumptions become particularly relevant in the application of this model to valvular disease and the right heart.

In contrast to the arterial pressure, the index of ventricular afterload, which is the product of arterial and ventricular properties, Ea provides a comprehensive description of those properties specific to the arterial system that oppose flow. Arterial impedance is independent of heart rate. However, because Ea is significantly influenced by heart rate, Ea is not a pure index of the arterial load. Figure 2.4 illustrates the effects of isolated changes in Ea on Pes and SV, and Figs. 2.5 and 2.6 illustrate the effects of changes in heart rate on Ea.

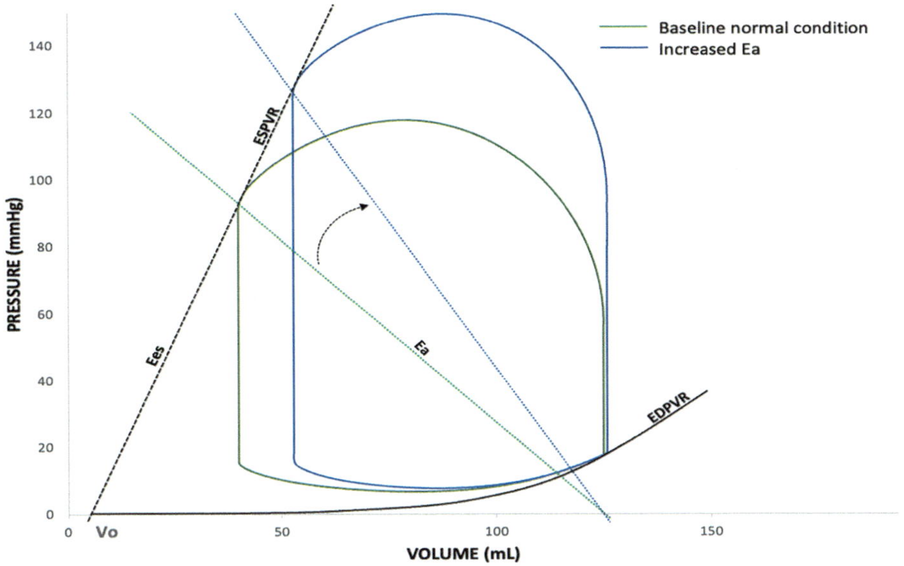

Fig. 2.4 *Alterations in arterial load.* Ventricular PVLs illustrating the impact of changes in Ea. The isolated increase in Ea (arterial load) has increased Ea/Ees, thus the EF and SV decrease. Pes has increased because Ea has increased and Ees is unchanged. Ventricular afterload (systolic BP) and the PVA have increased

The Pressure-Volume Area and Myocardial Oxygen Consumption

In addition to providing a construct for describing ventricular mechanics, the pressure-volume diagram provides a framework for understanding the determinants of myocardial VO_2. Frank was the first to characterize the external mechanical work (or stroke work, SW) performed by the ventricle to eject a SV as the area within the PVL (SW = Pes X SV) (Fig. 2.1). Suga and colleagues extended this concept by demonstrating a strong positive correlation between Frank's loop (SW) and the area of remaining mechanical potential energy (PE) at end systole (the area circumscribed by the EDPVR, ESPVR, and the diastolic portion of the PVL) (Fig. 2.1) and myocardial VO_2 [4]. The sum of SW and PE is the pressure-volume area (PVA), with the VO_2 cost per unit SW and unit PE being equal.

The PVA represents the total mechanical work resulting from actin-myosin cross-bridge cycling. Figure 2.7 illustrates the positive linear relationship between myocardial VO_2 and the PVA. There are also PVA independent determinants of VO_2, which are basal metabolism and the cost of calcium cycling associated with

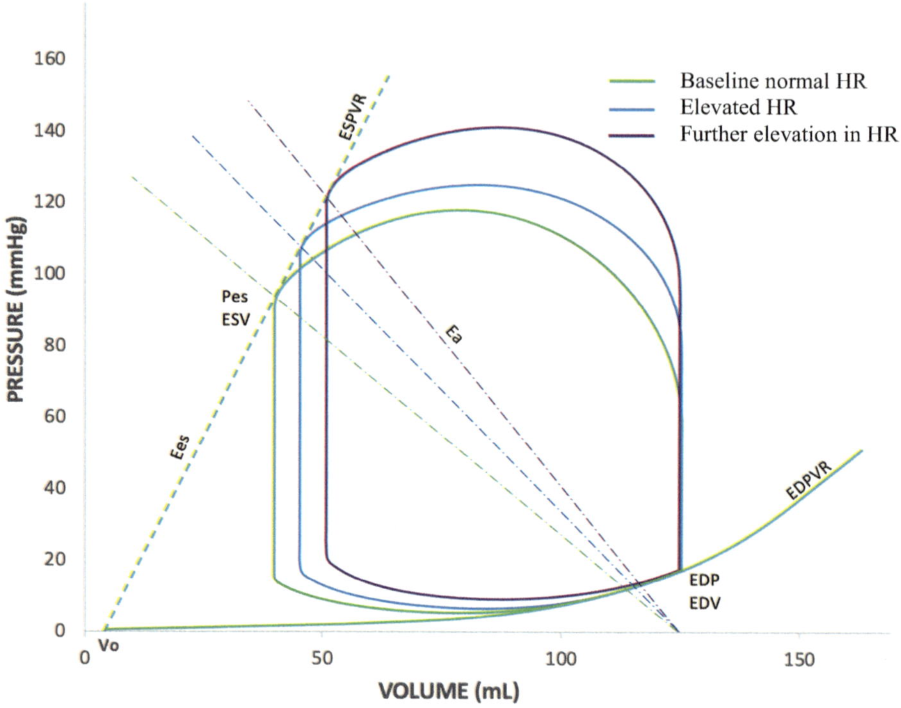

Fig. 2.5 *Impact of alterations in HR on the arterial load.* These ventricular PVLs illustrate the impact of increases in HR on effective Ea. In this instance, the EDV is maintained by increasing the SBV (see Chap. 5). Increases in HR increase effective Ea and the ratio of Pes/SV. Because Ea/Ees increases, the EF and SV decrease. The increase in HR increases LV afterload (systolic BP)

excitation-contraction-relaxation (ECR) (Fig. 2.7) [4]. An increase in calcium cycling, as occurs with inotropy, is reflected in an upward, parallel shift of the VO_2-PVA relationship (the hinge point shifts upward) (Fig. 2.7) [4]. The relationship between PVA-independent VO_2 and Ees is an indicator of the economy of contractility. For a given Ees, hypothermia and alkalosis decrease PVA-independent VO_2, while acidosis and hyperthermia increase it [4, 13]. Basal metabolism does not change significantly with changes in inotropy or ventricular loading conditions. Positive inotropy increases myocardial VO_2 in a PVA-dependent and independent manner. An increase in ventricular preload (EDV) and afterload (Ea) increases myocardial VO_2 in a PVA-dependent manner and does not affect ECR-related energy consumption [4, 13].

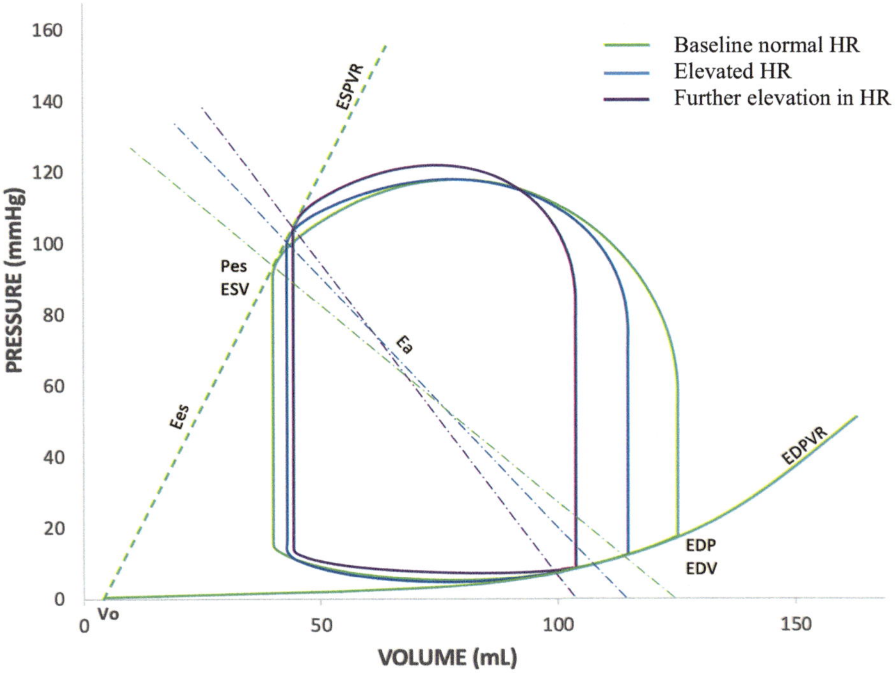

Fig. 2.6 *The impact of alterations in HR on ventricular loading conditions.* These PVLs illustrate the impact of isolated increases in HR on effective Ea. The increase in HR decreases the time for ventricular filling, and consequently the EDV, while increasing the Pes

Ventricular Arterial Coupling and Mechanical Efficiency

For a given preload, the relationship between Ea and Ees determines the degree of ventricular ejection (the ventricular ejection fraction [EF]), SV, and Pes. The normal ratio of Ea/Ees is approximately 0.6 for the systemic and pulmonary circulations [11, 14–17]. This ratio is inversely related to the EF and SV. For example, as the ratio increases, either due to an increase in Ea and/or decrease in Ees, the ventricle becomes uncoupled from its arterial system, and the EF and SV decrease. It is also important to consider absolute changes in Ea and Ees and their impact on Pes. If, for example, Ea and Ees increase to the same extent, EF and SV will remain the same; however, Pes will increase (Fig. 2.8).

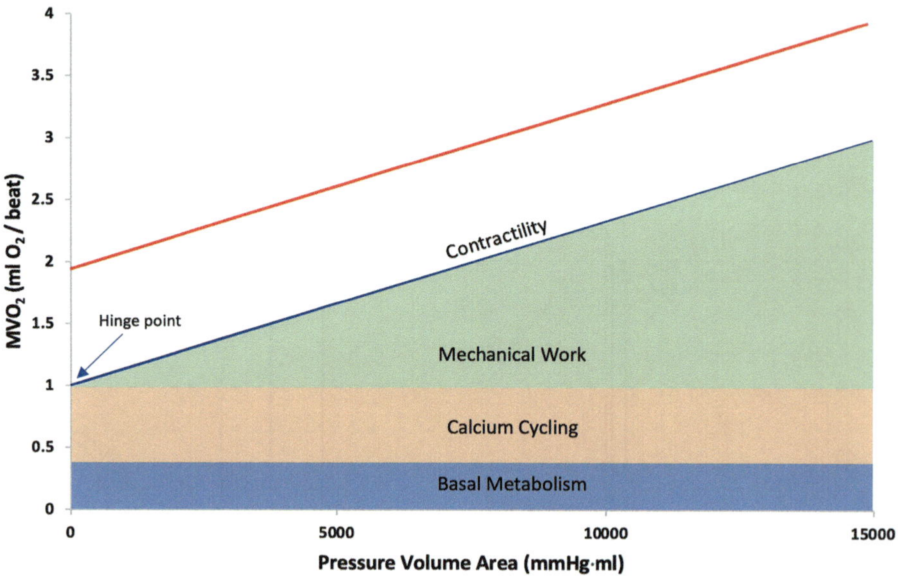

Fig. 2.7 *The relationship between PVA and myocardial VO_2 and the determinants of myocardial VO_2*. There is a positive linear relationship between actin-myosin cross-bridge cycling (mechanical work) and PVA and myocardial VO_2. Alterations in excitation-contraction-relaxation and calcium cycling affect myocardial VO_2 in a PVA-independent manner. An increase in calcium cycling, as occurs with positive inotropy, is reflected in an upward, parallel shift of the VO_2-PVA relationship (the hinge point shifts upward [red line])

The ratio of Ea/Ees also determines the efficiency of energy transfer from the ventricle to its arterial system. Burkhoff and Sagawa derived an analytical model relating the properties of the arterial system and ventricle to the mechanical work done by the heart and the amount of energy consumed by it [18]. Mechanical efficiency may be viewed as the amount of SW performed relative to the PVA (SW/PVA). Optimal mechanical efficiency occurs when Ees is nearly twice Ea (i.e., when Ea/Ees = 0.6) and results in the least amount of energy "wasted" as PE. As Ea increases and/or Ees decreases, the proportion of PE to the PVA increases, and as a result mechanical efficiency and the optimality of ventricular arterial coupling decrease.

Figures 2.3, 2.4, 2.5, 2.6, 2.8, and 2.9 illustrate the effects of changes in Ea, Ees, Ea/Ees, and EDV on SV, Pes, and mechanical efficiency. Figure 2.4 illustrates that for a given EDV and Ees, as Ea increases, Pes increases, and the EF and SV decrease. This conversion of volume work (SV) to pressure work (Pes) decreases mechanical

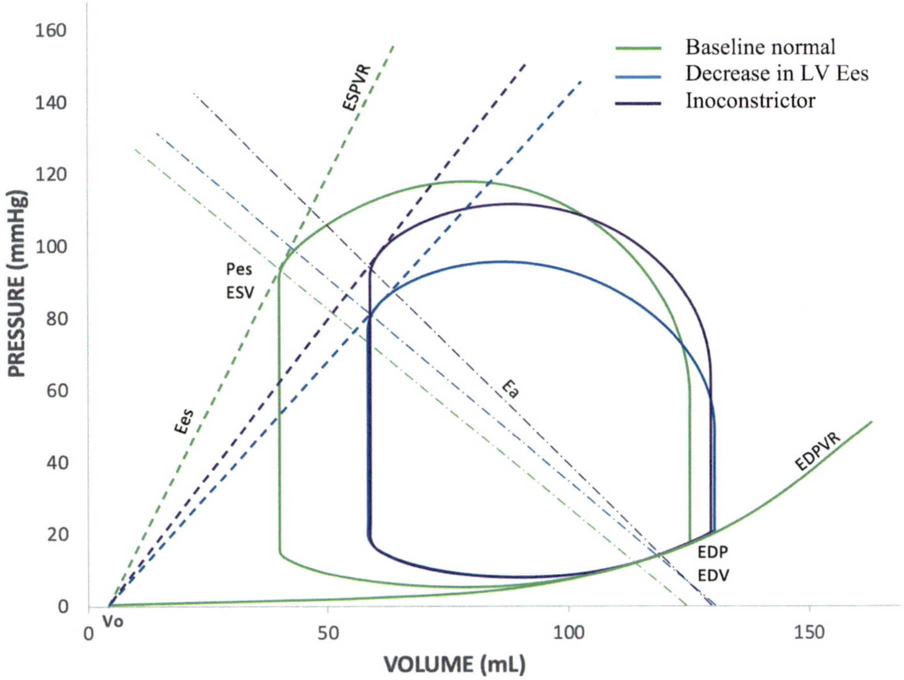

Fig. 2.8 *The impact of absolute and relative changes in ventricular and arterial elastance*. These PVLs illustrate the impact of a decrease in LV Ees followed by the effect of an inoconstrictor on the relationship between Ea and Ees. In this instance, the agent has increased Ea and Ees equally. As a result, Pes, as well as mean and systolic pressure, increase; however, because Ea/Ees remains the same, the EF and SV are unchanged

efficiency of the ventricle and is reflected by an increase in PE, PVA, and myocardial VO_2. Suga and colleagues demonstrated in isolated canine hearts that the heart performing a given SW consumes significantly more oxygen when ejection pressure is high, SV is small than when ejection pressure is lower, and SV is larger due to a greater PE and PVA in the pressure-loaded heart [19]. Figure 2.3 illustrates that for a given EDV and Ea, as Ees decreases, SW decreases as pressure (Pes) and flow work (SV) decrease. The proportion of the PVA that is PE increases and mechanical efficiency decreases. Whether due to an increase in Ea, decrease in Ees, or both, as the ventricle becomes uncoupled from its arterial system, and Ea/Ees rises above 0.5, PE increases, and mechanical efficiency, EF, and SV decrease. Figure 2.9 shows the effects of isolated changes in EDV.

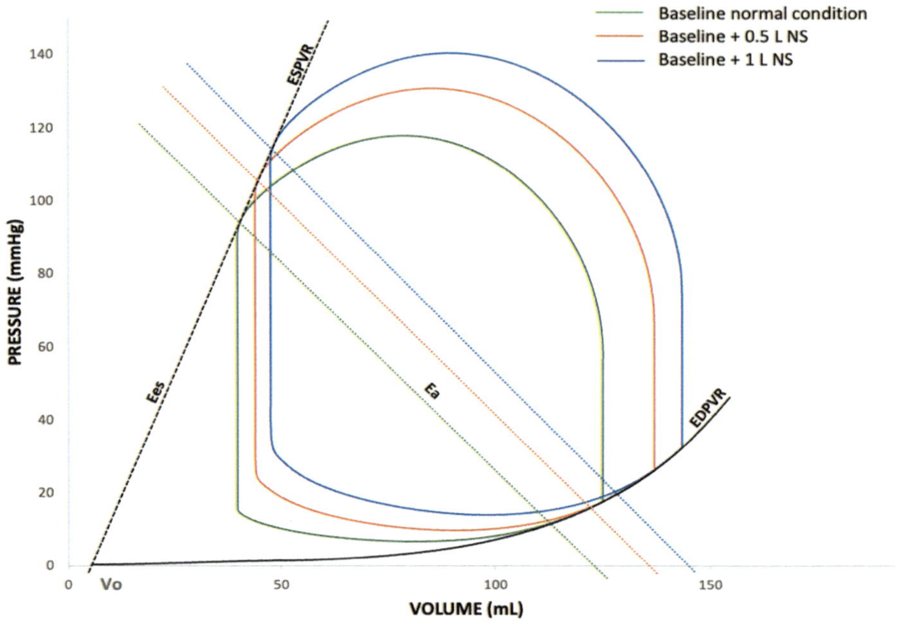

Fig. 2.9 *The impact of intravascular volume administration.* Ventricular PVLs illustrating the impact of isolated, sequential normal saline (NS) fluid boluses on SBV, systemic venous return, and ultimately LV EDV. With each 500 ml bolus, operating chamber stiffness increases, the resulting incremental change in EDV decreases, reflecting volume-dependent changes in chamber stiffness. The arterial load Ea is unaffected but ventricular afterload, the systolic BP (as well as the ventricular systolic radius), and PVA have increased. The EF is insensitive to changes in preload [20, 21]. The primary determinant of the EF is Ea/Ees [21]

Conclusion

The work of Suga and Sunagawa and others provides an approach for modeling the complete cardiovascular system and in doing so provides a basis for understanding, simulating, and illustrating cardiovascular physiology and pathophysiology and the impact of therapies.

References

1. Kuhtz-Buschbeck JP, Drake-Holland A, Noble MIM, et al. Rediscovery of Otto Frank's contribution to science. J Mol Cell Cardiol. 2018;119:96–103.
2. Suga H, Sagawa K. Instantaneous pressure-volume relationships and their ratio in the excised, supported canine left ventricle. Circ Res. 1974;35:117–26.
3. Sunagawa K, Maughan L, Burkhoff D, et al. Left ventricular interaction with arterial load studied in isolated canine ventricle. Am J Phys. 1983;245:H773–80.

4. Suga H. Total mechanical energy of a ventricle model and cardiac oxygen consumption. Am J Phys. 1979;236:H498–505.
5. Burkhoff D, Mirsky I, Suga H. Assessment of systolic and diastolic ventricular properties via pressure-volume analysis: a guide for clinical, translational, and basic researchers. Am J Physiol Heart Circ Physiol. 2005;289:H501–12.
6. Zile MR, Brutsaert DL. New concepts in diastolic dysfunction and diastolic heart failure: part I: diagnosis, prognosis, and measurements of diastolic function. Circulation. 2002;105:1387–93.
7. Glantz SA, Parmley WW. Factors which affect the diastolic pressure-volume curve. Circ Res. 1978;42:171–80.
8. Mirsky I, Pasipoularides A. Clinical assessment of diastolic function. Prog Cardiovasc Dis. 1990;32:291–318.
9. Gaasch WH. Left ventricular radius to wall thickness ratio. Am J Cardiol. 1979;43:1189–94.
10. Gaasch WH, Levine HJ, Quinones MA, et al. Left ventricular compliance: mechanisms and clinical implications. Am J Cardiol. 1976;38:645–53.
11. Sunagawa K, Sagawa K, Maughan WL. Ventricular interaction with the loading system. Ann Biomed Eng. 1984;12:163–89.
12. Kelly RP, Ting C-T, Yang T-M, et al. Effective arterial elastance as index of arterial vascular load in humans. Circulation. 1992;86:513–21.
13. Suga H. Global cardiac function: mechano-energetico-informatics. J Biomech. 2003;36:713–20.
14. Nevo E. Constrained optimization of ventricular efficiency in normal and failing hearts. Am J Phys. 1993;264:H1292–9.
15. Sasayama S, Asanoi H. Coupling between the heart and arterial system in heart failure. Am J Med. 1991;90(suppl 5B):5B–15S.
16. Little WC, Pu M. Left ventricular-arterial coupling. J Am Soc Echocardiogr. 2009;22:1246–8.
17. Chantler PD, Lakatta EG, Najjar SS. Arterial-ventricular coupling: mechanistic insights into cardiovascular performance at rest and during exercise. J Appl Physiol. 2008;105:1342–51.
18. Burkhoff D, Sagawa K. Ventricular efficiency predicted by an analytical model. Am J Phys. 1986;250:R1021–7.
19. Suga H, Hisano R, Hirata S, et al. Mechanism of higher oxygen consumption rate: pressure-loaded vs. volume-loaded heart. Am J Phys. 1982;242:H942–8.
20. Robotham JL, Takata M, Berman M, et al. Ejection fraction revisited. Anesthesiology. 1991;74:172–83.
21. Kass DA, Lowell Maughan W, Guo ZM, et al. Comparative influence of load versus inotropic states on indexes of ventricular contractility: experimental and theoretical analysis based on pressure-volume relationships. Circulation. 1987;6:1422–36.

Chapter 3
Diastolic Function and Dysfunction

Ronald A. Bronicki and Daniel J. Penny

Diastolic dysfunction contributes importantly to the pathophysiology of many diseases commonly encountered in the critical care setting and is associated with adverse outcomes [1–4].

Diastolic function may be viewed as the ability of the ventricle to fill. Diastolic dysfunction results from an abnormality in ventricular relaxation or distensibility, both of which may contribute to an impairment in ventricular filling. Diastolic heart failure therefore may be considered a state in which the ventricle is unable to accept an adequate volume, at normal diastolic pressure and at volumes sufficient to maintain an adequate stroke volume [5].

Myocardial relaxation is the process by which the myocardium returns to an unstressed length and force. As calcium is extruded from the cytosol and myofilament cross-bridges detach, myocardial tension is quickly reduced, and ventricular pressure falls rapidly. Thus, the fall in ventricular pressure is the hemodynamic manifestation of myocardial relaxation. Under normal conditions, relaxation begins during late ejection, continues throughout the isovolumic phase of the cardiac cycle, and concludes during the period of rapid filling. Impaired relaxation is characterized by cross-bridge cycling and tone extending further into the filling phase than normal, adversely affecting the onset, rate, and extent of decline in ventricular pressure and, in turn, ventricular filling.

Several measures of ventricular relaxation have been derived by examining a mathematical function of its pressure decay [5–8]. One such measure is the parameter tau, the exponential time constant of pressure decay, where tau is the time it takes for ventricular pressure to fall to 1/e (~36%) of its initial value and where complete relaxation occurs over approximately 3.5-time constants after aortic valve closure. On the ventricular pressure volume loop, impaired relaxation is reflected in

R. A. Bronicki (✉) · D. J. Penny
Baylor College of Medicine, Texas Children's Hospital, Houston, TX, USA
e-mail: rxbronic@texaschildrens.org; djpenny@texaschildrens.org

R. A. Bronicki et al. (eds.), *Simulation in Cardiovascular Critical Care Medicine*, https://doi.org/10.1007/978-3-031-63557-1_3

an upward shift of the diastolic pressure volume relationship (Figs. 3.1, 3.2, and 3.3) [8, 9]. Incomplete relaxation is reflected in the end diastolic pressure volume coordinate not reaching the end diastolic pressure volume relationship (EDPVR) (Figs. 3.2 and 3.3) [9].

Myocardial relaxation is modulated by myofilament inactivation, ventricular load, and nonuniformity. Inactivation occurs in a series of energy-consuming steps beginning with the dissociation of calcium from troponin C, detachment of the actin-myosin cross-bridge, phosphorylation of phospholamban, sarcoplasmic reticulum calcium ATPase pump (SERCA)-induced calcium resequestration into the sarcoplasmic reticulum, and the extrusion of calcium from the cytoplasm across the sarcolemma. For these reasons, adequate energy is needed for this process to occur at a sufficient rate and extent. Other mechanisms related to calcium homeostasis may also affect myocardial inactivation. Decrease concentration or activity of SERCA can slow the removal of cytosolic calcium. Decreased SERCA activity is seen in concentric hypertrophy and dilated and hypertrophic cardiomyopathies.

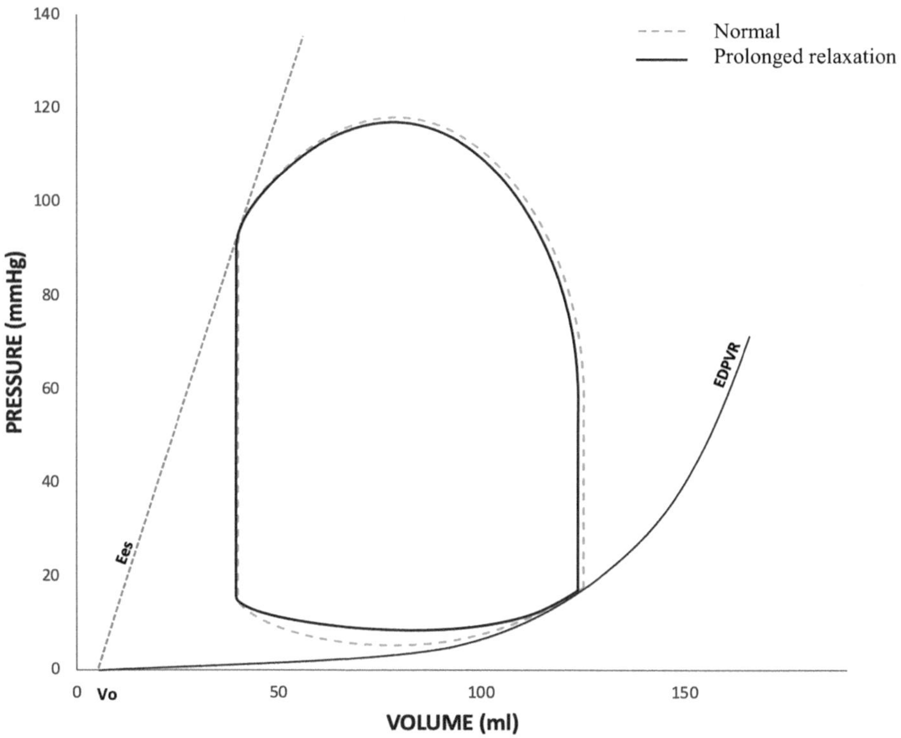

Fig. 3.1 *Normal and prolonged ventricular relaxation.* These PVLs illustrate the impact of a nearly four-fold increase in tau with a HR of 60. Impaired relaxation is reflected in the upward shift in the diastolic pressure volume relationship. Despite a significant prolongation of LV relaxation, there is no appreciable effect on the LV EDV and thus EDP. Ventricular relaxation is completed and is reflected in the end diastolic pressure volume coordinate reaching the EDPVR

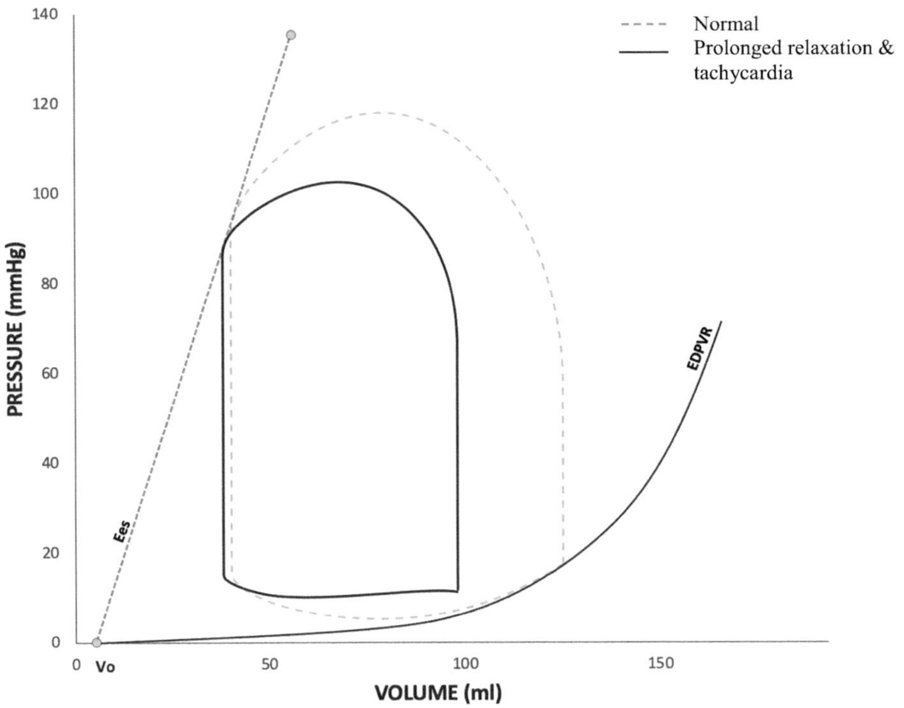

Fig. 3.2 *The impact of prolonged ventricular relaxation coupled with tachycardia.* These PVLs illustrate that prolonged LV relaxation (unchanged from Fig. 3.1) coupled with tachycardia (HR has increased from 60 to 85) leads to incomplete relaxation, which is indicated by the end diastolic pressure volume coordinate not reaching the EDPVR. Prolonged relaxation coupled with tachycardia leads to a significant decrease in the EDV. In this case, the EDP has decreased while the mean left atrial pressure (PAOP) has increased

Increased levels or activity of phospholamban, a SERCA-inhibitory protein, impairs relaxation. Increased cAMP, resulting from beta adrenergic stimulation or inhibition of cardiac phosphodiesterase, phosphorylates phospholamban, decreasing its inhibitory effect on SERCA. Additional determinants of myocardial inactivation include alterations in myofilaments that affect their interaction or calcium sensitivity.

Myocardial relaxation is also dependent on ventricular loading conditions and uniformity of activation [10]. Changes in ventricular load will alter cross-bridge formation during systole and, in turn, also effect relaxation. The precise alterations will depend on the type of load (volume versus pressure) and its duration and timing in the cardiac cycle [10]. The clinical significance of this in vivo is unclear [10]. In various pathologic conditions such as conduction disturbances, ischemic or infarcted muscle, and cardiomyopathies, nonuniformity in activation leads to regional mechanical asynchrony that adversely affects not only contraction but also myocardial relaxation.

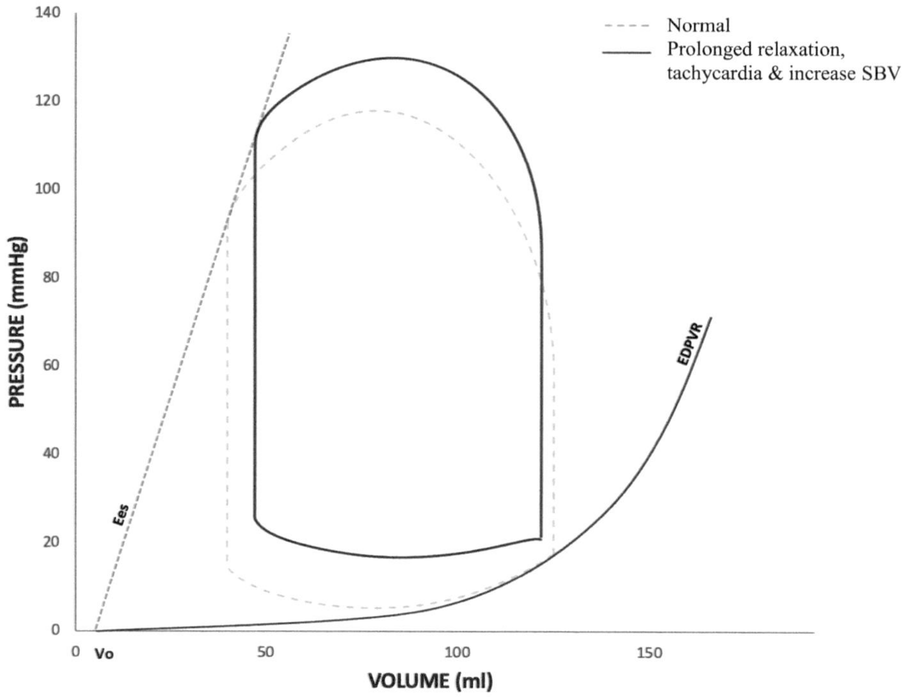

Fig. 3.3 *Prolonged ventricular relaxation coupled with tachycardia and an increase in SBV.* These PVLs illustrate the impact of prolonged ventricular relaxation and tachycardia accompanied by an increase in SBV (see Chap. 5) and pulmonary venous pressure such that the extent of LV filling approaches normal. As a result, the marked decrease in LV distensibility is now reflected in a significantly elevated EDP. Ventricular relaxation remains incompleteUnder normal conditions, the mean left atrial pressure (PAOP) and LV EDP are similar in magnitude. However, a marked impairment in ventricular relaxation influences the mean left atrial pressure to a greater effect than the EDP. In this case, the mean left atrial pressure increased by 12 and the EDP by 4 mmHg, respectively

If the rate of ventricular filling is impaired in mid- and early diastole because of an abnormality of ventricular relaxation, it is then essential that the ventricle has adequate time to compensate for this deficiency during late diastole. As a result, the clinical setting in which relaxation delay influences diastolic pressure and ventricular filling the most is tachycardia (Figs. 3.1, 3.2, and 3.3) [9]. Tachycardia not only influences myocardial oxygen demand and coronary perfusion time but may shorten diastole to an extent that prevents complete relaxation between beats. The effects of alterations in myocardial relaxation on left ventricular diastolic pressure and volume with a range of heart rates are illustrated in Figs. 3.1, 3.2, and 3.3.

The other determinant of ventricular diastolic function is chamber stiffness. Chamber stiffness is a function of geometry and the material properties of the myocardium [5, 6, 11]. The EDPVR reflects the cumulative effect of geometric and material properties and indicates ventricular stiffness or compliance (the inverse of stiffness). A shift of the EDPVR curve upward and leftward is indicative of an increase in stiffness (Figs. 3.4, 3.5, and 3.6). In this case, a greater diastolic transmural pressure is required to generate the same end diastolic volume as a normal ventricle. A shift downward and rightward is indicative of a decrease in stiffness. The EDPVR is nonlinear, a characteristic attributed to the different types of structural fibers being stretched. For a given EDPVR, as volume increases, the pressure begins to rise, and with large volume, the pressure increases disproportionately. That is to say that *operating chamber stiffness* increases at higher volumes (volume-dependent changes in chamber stiffness) [5, 6, 11].

Alterations in chamber geometry affect chamber stiffness and result from changes in the ventricular muscle mass or wall thickness to end diastolic volume ratio, with stiffness varying directly with this ratio [11–17]. Alterations in ventricular geometry result from either physiological or pathological ventricular remodeling. Physiologic hypertrophy, as seen with exercise, increases equally the muscle mass and chamber volume, and thus there is no change in ventricular stiffness. A diastolic volume load resulting from mitral regurgitation, for example, stimulates

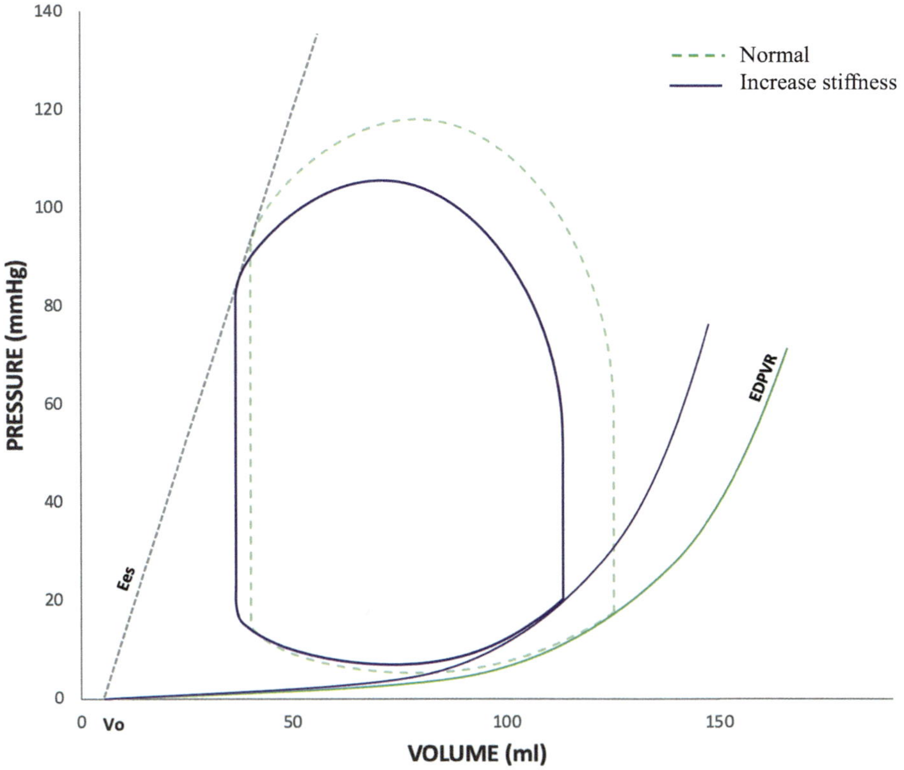

Fig. 3.4 *Elevated LV stiffness.* These PVLs illustrate the impact of a significant increase in LV stiffness. The EDPVR is shifted up and to the left. Without changing any other parameter, the EDV is reduced. As a result, the mean left atrial pressure (PAOP) and EDP are minimally elevated

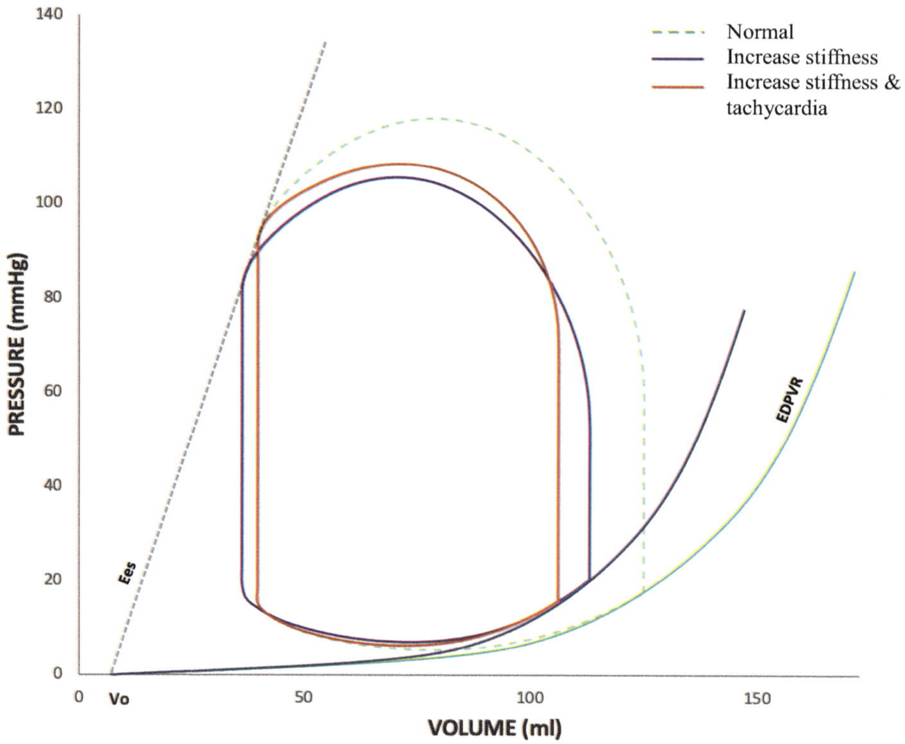

Fig. 3.5 *Increase LV stiffness and tachycardia.* These PVLs illustrate the effect of the same degree of increase in LV stiffness as in Fig. 3.4 coupled with tachycardia (HR has increased from 60 to 85). The EDV and thus EDP have decreased further

structural remodeling of the left ventricle, resulting in an increase in left ventricular capacitance. If left ventricular volume increases to a greater degree than the associated compensatory increase in wall thickness, left ventricular stiffness decreases. A systolic pressure load resulting from aortic stenosis, for example, leads to concentric hypertrophy. The resulting increase in the ventricular mass-to-volume ratio increases chamber stiffness. Eccentric remodeling as seen in chronic systolic heart failure is characterized by a marked increase in chamber volume with little to no increase in muscle mass. As a result, chamber stiffness is significantly reduced. Acute changes in ventricular geometry may occur following interventions for valvular disease as well [18]. The hemodynamic impact of ventricular remodeling and acute changes in ventricular geometry are covered in detail with specific lesions elsewhere in this book.

Myocardial stiffness refers to the intrinsic properties of the myocardium and is reflected in the myocardial stress-strain relationship, the resistance of the myocardium to stretch when subjected to stress [11]. Alterations in myocardial properties result from changes in the cardiomyocyte and/or extracellular matrix. Changes in the composition of the cardiomyocyte cytoskeleton may alter ventricular stiffness.

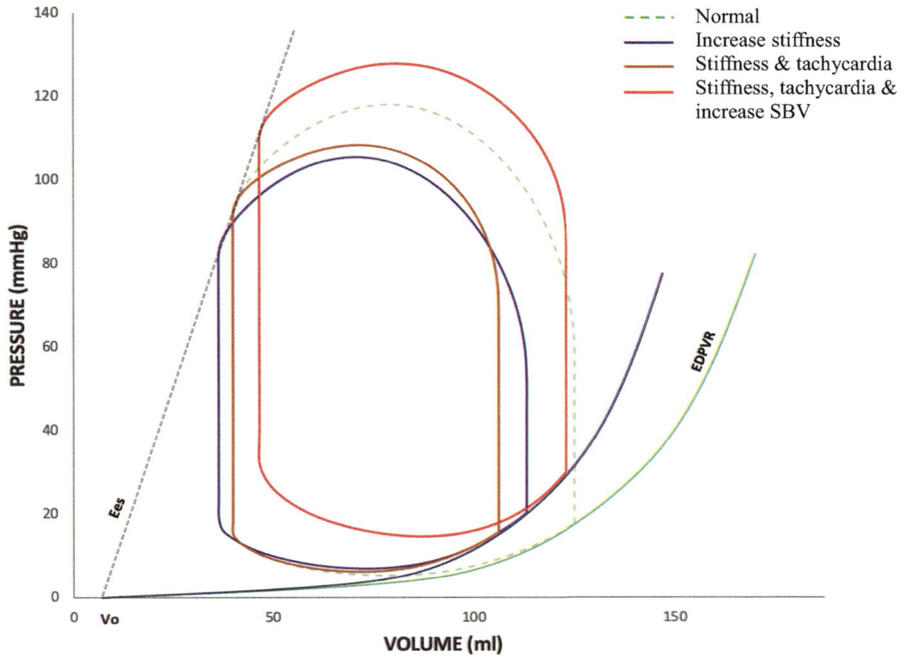

Fig. 3.6 *Increase LV stiffness coupled with tachycardia and an increase in SBV.* These PVLs illustrate the impact of the same increase in LV stiffness as in Figs. 3.4 and 3.5 coupled with tachycardia and now a compensatory increase in the SBV such that the LV EDV approaches the baseline, normal value. The mean left atrial pressure (PAOP) and EDP are now significantly elevated at 28 and 30 mmHg, respectively

Changes in the sarcomeric protein titin, for example, not only effect stiffness but also relaxation. Changes in the composition of the extracellular matrix can affect ventricular stiffness, most importantly alterations in collagen. Importantly, acute changes in stiffness may result from inflammation-induced edema. Activation of inflammatory pathways is essential to the pathophysiology of myocardial ischemia-reperfusion injury and cardiopulmonary bypass-induced myocardial dysfunction. Sepsis and myocarditis also induce edema [1–4, 19–26] (Figs. 3.7 and 3.8).

Other factors external to the heart may alter the effective compliance of the entire heart. Changes in intrathoracic pressure alter the surrounding pressure of the heart, the diastolic transmural pressure, and the effective compliance for each chamber. The extent to which this occurs depends on the magnitude of change in airway pressure and the extent to which this change in airway pressure is transmitted to the cardiac fossa (see Chap. 5 on heart lung interactions). Elevated right ventricular diastolic pressure decreases the normal transeptal pressure gradient, causing it to deviate into the left ventricle, decreasing the effective compliance of the left ventricle. Pericardial disease alters the effective compliance of the heart; the extent to which this occurs depends in part on the rate of development and the magnitude of the lesion.

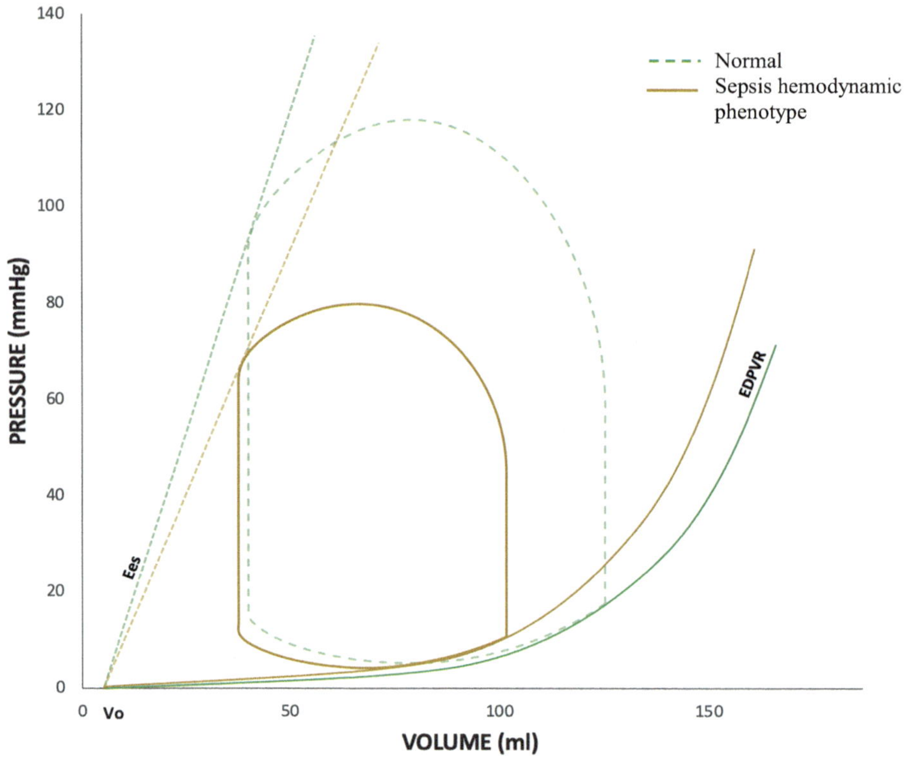

Fig. 3.7 *Diastolic dysfunction in sepsis.* These PVLs illustrate changes consistent with a hemodynamic phenotype of sepsis characterized by a decrease in LV contractility (Ees) and vascular tone. SVR and Ea are decreased (not shown). Venomotor tone and SBV are reduced, which coupled with an acute increase in ventricular stiffness due to inflammation-induced LV edema, leading to a decrease in EDV. Despite the presence of impaired LV diastolic function, the EDP is not elevated

The assessment of diastolic function may be divided into those that reflect the process of active relaxation and those that reflect passive stiffness. Doppler echocardiography may be used to assess transmitral and pulmonary venous flow patterns. These measurements however are often difficult to obtain in critically ill patients and are influenced by loading conditions.

In the following simulations, we illustrate the physiology of diastolic function and the pathophysiology and clinical relevance of diastolic dysfunction.

Conclusion

Diastolic dysfunction contributes importantly to the pathophysiology of many diseases commonly encountered in the critical care setting and is associated with adverse outcomes. In this review we have discussed diastolic function and

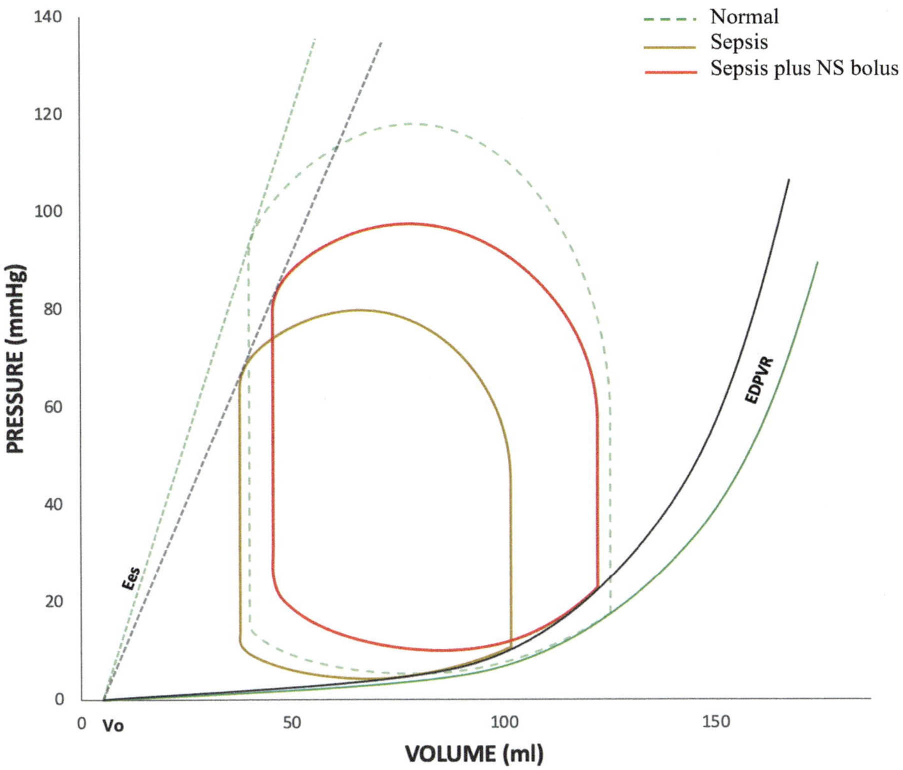

Fig. 3.8 *Diastolic dysfunction coupled with intravascular volume in sepsis.* These PVLs illustrate the hemodynamic phenotype of sepsis described in Fig. 3.7 and the impact of the administration of 40 cc/kg of normal saline (NS). The LV EDV approaches the baseline, normal value. However, fluid resuscitation has increased the LV EDP considerably causing hydrostatic pulmonary edema

illustrated the pathophysiology and clinical relevance of diastolic dysfunction and failure.

References

1. Sanfilippo F, Scolletta S, Morelli A, et al. Practical approach to diastolic dysfunction in light of the new guidelines and clinical applications in the operating room and in the intensive are. Ann Intensive Care. 2018;8:100.
2. Sanfilippo F, Corredor C, Fletcher N, et al. Diastolic dysfunction and mortality in septic patients: a systematic review and meta-analysis. Intensive Care Med. 2015;41:1004–13.
3. Godfrey GEP, Peck MJE. Diastolic dysfunction in anaesthesia and critical care. BJA Educ. 2016;9:287–91.
4. Lanspa MJ, Gutsche AR, Wilson EL, et al. Application of a simplified definition of diastolic function in severe sepsis and septic shock. Crit Care. 2016;20:243.

5. Zile MR, Brutsaert DL. New concepts in diastolic dysfunction and diastolic heart failure: Part I: diagnosis, prognosis, and measurements of diastolic function. Circulation. 2002;105:1387–93.
6. Zile MR, Brutsaert DL. New concepts in diastolic dysfunction and diastolic heart failure: Part II: causal mechanisms and treatment. Circulation. 2002;105:1503–8.
7. Leite-Moreira AF. Diastolic dysfunction and diastolic heart failure. Heart. 2006;92:712–8.
8. Burkhoff D, Maurer MS, Packer M. Heart failure with a normal ejection fraction. Is it really a disorder of diastolic function? Circulation. 2003;107:656–8.
9. Hay I, Rich J, Ferber P, et al. Role of impaired myocardial relaxation in the production of elevated left ventricular filling pressure. Am J Physiol Heart Circ Physiol. 2005;288:H1203–8.
10. Kass DA, Bronzwaer JGF, Paulus WJ. What mechanisms underlie diastolic dysfunction in heart failure? Circ Res. 2004;94:1533–42.
11. Burkhoff D, Mirsky I, Suga H. Assessment of systolic and diastolic ventricular properties via pressure-volume analysis: a guide for clinical, translational, and basic researchers. Am J Physiol Heart Circ Physiol. 2005;289:H501–12.
12. Litwin SE, Grossman W. Diastolic dysfunction as a cause of heart failure. J Am Coll Cardiol. 1993;4(Suppl A):49A–55A.
13. Mandinov L, Eberli FR, Seiler C, et al. Review diastolic heart failure. Cardiovasc Res. 2000;45:813–25.
14. Glantz SA, Parmley WW. Factors which affect the diastolic pressure-volume curve. Circ Res. 1978;42:171–80.
15. Grossman W, Paulus WJ. Myocardial stress and hypertrophy: a complex interface between biophysics and cardiac remodeling. J Clin Invest. 2013;123:3701–3.
16. Gaasch WH, Levine HJ, Quiniones MA, et al. Left ventricular compliance: mechanism and clinical implications. Am J Cardiol. 1976;38:645–53.
17. Gaasch WH, Zile MR. Left ventricular structural remodeling in health and disease. With special emphasis on volume, mass, and geometry. J Am Coll Cardiol. 2011;58:1733–40.
18. Zaid RR, Barker CM, Little SH, et al. Pre- and post-operative diastolic dysfunction in patients with valvular heart disease. J Am Coll Cardiol. 2013;62:1922–30.
19. Blatchford JW III, Barragry TP, Lillehei T, et al. Effects of cardioplegic arrest on left ventricular systolic and diastolic function of the intact neonatal heart. J Thorac Cardiovasc Surg. 1994;107:527–35.
20. Egan JR, Butler TL, Cole AD, et al. Myocardial ischemia is more important than the effects of cardiopulmonary bypass on myocardial water handling and postoperative dysfunction: a pediatric animal model. J Thorac Cardiovasc Surg. 2008;136:1265–73.
21. Hsu DT, Weng Z-C, Nicolosi AC, et al. Quantitative effects of myocardial edema on the left ventricular pressure-volume relation. J Thorac Cardiovasc Surg. 1993;106:651–7.
22. Nishio R, Sasayama S, Matsumori A. Left ventricular pressure-volume relationship in a murine model of congestive heart failure due to acute viral myocarditis. J Am Coll Cardiol. 2002;40:1506–14.
23. Tschope C, Westermann D, Steendijk P, et al. Hemodynamic characterization of left ventricular function in experimental coxsackie viral myocarditis: effects of carvedilol and metoprolol. Eur J Pharmacol. 2004;491:173–9.
24. Lauer B, Schannwell M, Kuhl U, et al. Antimyosin autoantibodies are associated with deterioration of systolic and diastolic left ventricular function in patient with chronic myocarditis. J Am Coll Cardiol. 2000;35:11–8.
25. Kakihana Y, Ito T, Nakahara M, et al. Sepsis-induced myocardial dysfunction: pathophysiology and management. J Intensive Care. 2016;4:22.
26. Walley KR. Sepsis-induced myocardial dysfunction. Curr Opin Crit Care. 2018;24(4):292–9.

Chapter 4
Determinants of Myocardial Oxygen Consumption and Delivery

Ronald A. Bronicki and Daniel J. Penny

Introduction

An understanding of the determinants of myocardial oxygen consumption (VO_2) and delivery (DO_2) is essential for understanding the pathophysiological basis and management of cardiovascular disease.

Determinants of Myocardial VO_2

The ventricular pressure volume relationship and the time-varying elastance model provide a framework for discussing the determinants of myocardial VO_2 [1]. These concepts are discussed in detail in Chap. 2.

There are pressure volume area (PVA)-dependent and PVA-independent determinants of myocardial VO_2 (Figs. 4.1 and 4.2) [2, 3]. The PVA represents the total mechanical work resulting from actin myosin cross-bridge cycling and is strongly and positively correlated with changes in myocardial VO_2 (Fig. 4.1). The PVA is composed of an area representing the external mechanical work or stroke work (the product of pressure work [end systolic pressure] and volume work [stroke volume]) performed by the ventricle plus the area of remaining mechanical energy (potential energy) at end systole (Fig. 4.1).

The PVA-independent determinants of myocardial VO_2 are basal metabolism and calcium cycling associated with excitation, contraction, and relaxation (ECR) (Fig. 4.2). Basal metabolism does not change significantly with changes in inotropy or ventricular loading conditions.

R. A. Bronicki (✉) · D. J. Penny
Baylor College of Medicine, Texas Children's Hospital, Houston, TX, USA
e-mail: rxbronic@texaschildrens.org; djpenny@texaschildrens.org

R. A. Bronicki et al. (eds.), *Simulation in Cardiovascular Critical Care Medicine*, https://doi.org/10.1007/978-3-031-63557-1_4

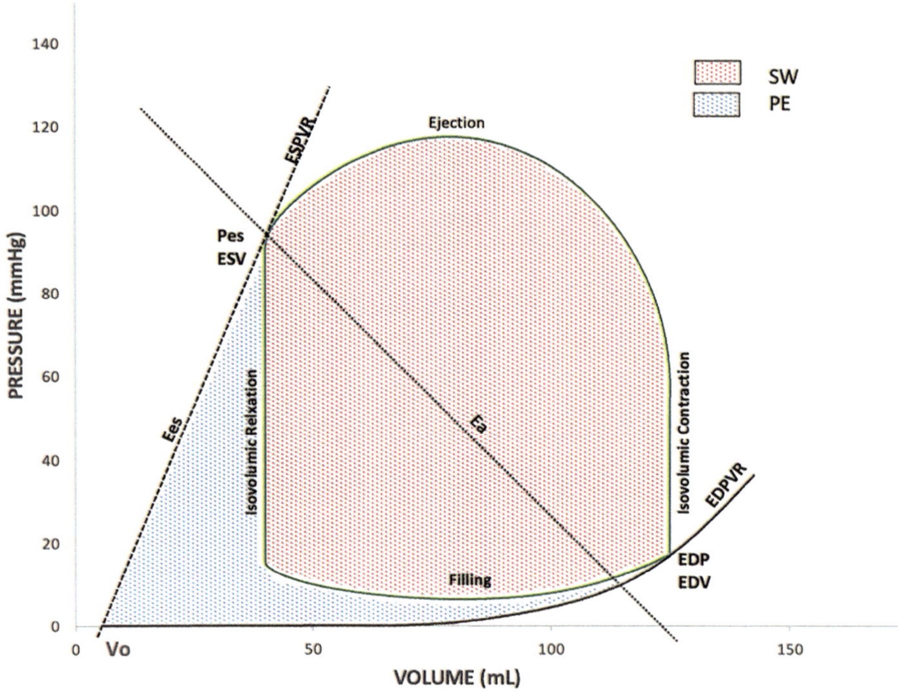

Fig. 4.1 *The ventricular PVL and the PVA-dependent determinants of myocardial VO_2.* The PVA is composed of SW, the product of pressure work (Pes) and volume work (SV), and PE, the mechanical energy remaining at end systole

Therapeutic Interventions and Myocardial VO_2

Positive inotropy increases myocardial VO_2 in a PVA-independent manner by increasing calcium cycling, reflected in an upward parallel shift of the PVA-VO_2 relationship (the hinge point shifts upward) (Fig. 4.2), and a PVA-dependent manner by increasing stroke work (pressure and stroke volume). Increasing ventricular preload (end diastolic volume) increases myocardial VO_2 in a PVA-dependent manner [1, 2]. An increase in the end diastolic volume increases myofilament sensitivity to calcium but does not alter contractility and thus does not alter ECR-related VO_2 [1, 2]. Increasing the arterial load (arterial elastance, Ea) increases myocardial VO_2 in a PVA-dependent manner [1, 2]. As Ea increases, the end systolic pressure (Pes) increases, and the ejection fraction and stroke volume decrease (Fig. 4.3). This conversion of volume work (stroke volume) to pressure work (Pes) decreases mechanical efficiency of the ventricle and is reflected by not only an increase in the PVA and myocardial VO_2 but also an increase in potential energy (Fig. 4.3). Suga and colleagues demonstrated in isolated canine hearts that the heart performing a given stroke work consumes significantly more oxygen when ejection pressure is high, and stroke volume is small than when ejection pressure is lower, and stroke volume

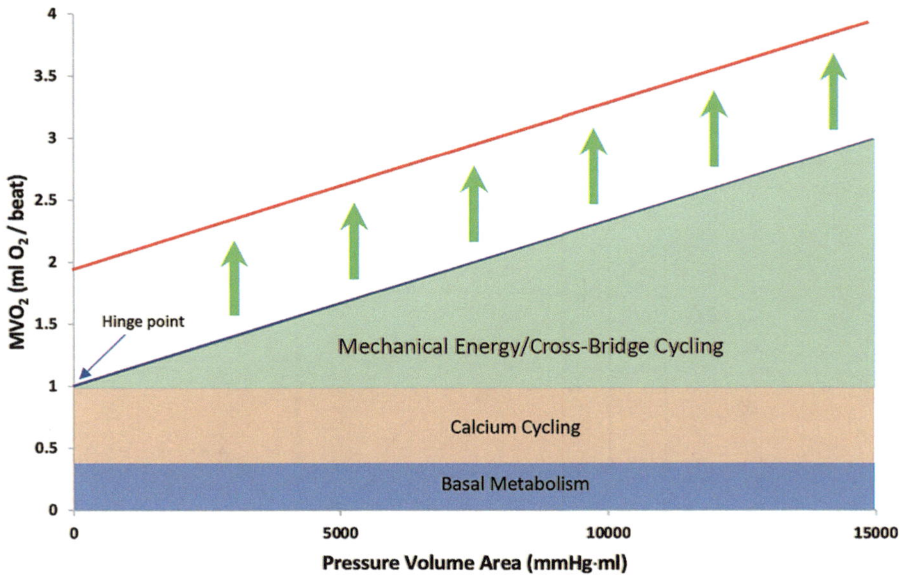

Fig. 4.2 *The determinants of myocardial* VO_2. The PVA is strongly and positively correlated with changes in myocardial VO_2. Inotropy affects calcium cycling. An increase in contractility (Ees) results in an increase in calcium cycling and is reflected in an upward, parallel shift of the PVA-myocardial VO_2 relationship and an upward shift in the hinge point. Calcium cycling and basal metabolism are PVA-independent determinants of myocardial VO_2

is larger due to a greater potential energy and PVA in the pressure-loaded heart [2, 3]. Elevations in heart rate increase Ea and arterial pressure and thus the PVA and myocardial VO_2 per minute, with marked elevations in heart rate by increasing contractility and ECR-related VO_2 [1, 2]. Lastly, muscle mass effects myocardial VO_2.

Determinants of Myocardial DO_2

Myocardial oxygen extraction at rest is upwards of 60–70%. Thus, the ability of an increase in oxygen extraction to maintain adequate myocardial oxygenation in the setting of an increase in oxygen demand, or decrease in DO_2, is limited. As a result, an increase in oxygen demand is dependent upon a corresponding increase in coronary flow. Under normal conditions, right ventricular (RV) perfusion results from the pressure gradient between the coronary arteries and right atrium. It is different for the left ventricle (LV), where coronary blood flow is characterized by marked variations during the cardiac cycle, the result of elevated myocardial tissue pressure and compression of the coronary microcirculatory vessels during systole [4–8].

The physical properties that govern the flow of fluids (liquid or air) through conducting passages, such as a vessel, are based on the general laws of hydrodynamics

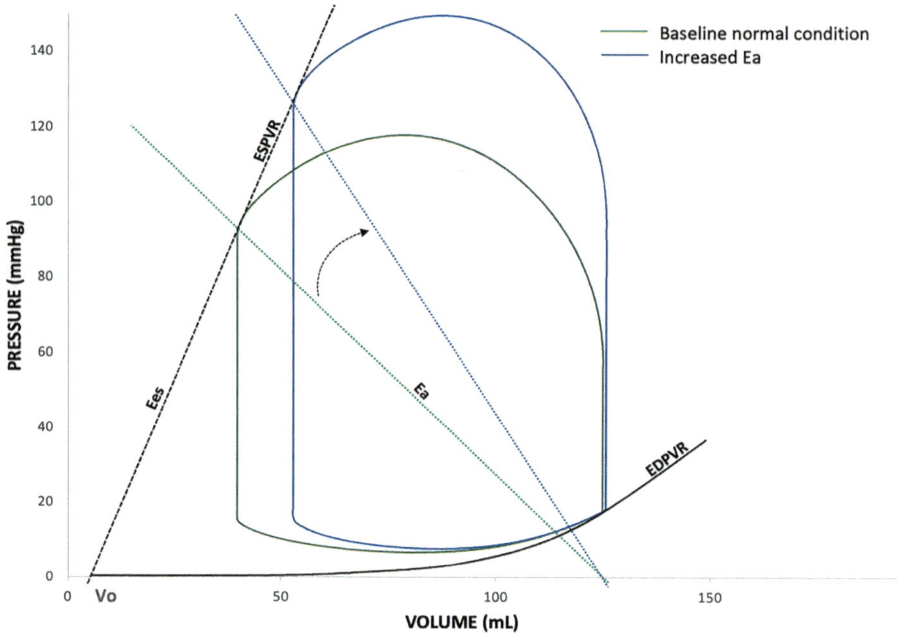

Fig. 4.3 *The impact of alterations in arterial load on myocardial* VO_2. Ventricular PVLs illustrating the impact of an isolated increase in Ea on the PVA, as well as SW, PE, and mechanical efficiency

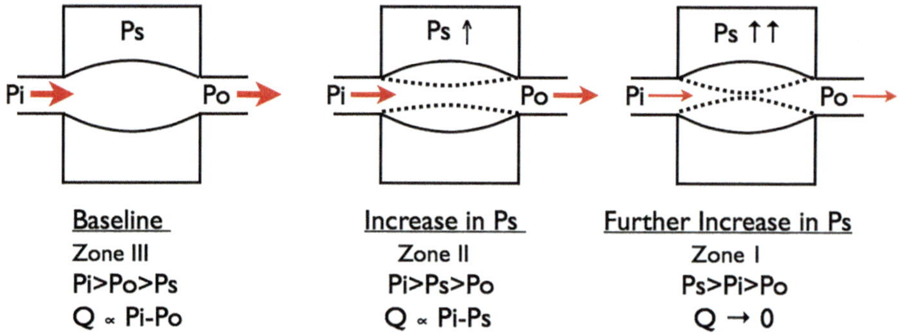

Fig. 4.4 *The laws of hydrodynamics applied to the coronary circulation.* Pi, Po, and Ps represent inlet, outlet, and surrounding pressure, respectively. At low Ps, the magnitude of flow through the tube is principally governed by the difference between Pi and Po (zone III conditions). If Ps is increased above Po, resistance to flow has increased and flow is governed by the difference between Pi and Ps (zone II conditions). Further increases in Ps to levels greater than Pi result in cessation of flow

(Fig. 4.4) [5, 6]. The behavior of flow (Q) through a collapsible structure depends on the inflow pressure (Pi = coronary artery pressure), outflow pressure (Po = right atrial pressure), the surrounding pressure (Ps = interstitial pressure), the vascular transmural pressure (Ptm = the difference between luminal and interstitial or surrounding pressure), and the compliance of the structure (Fig. 4.4). When the Ptm throughout the structure is positive, the tube is widely patent, and Q is proportional to the pressure gradient Pi—Po (also known as zone III conditions). With a constant Pi and Po, as the Ps increases, the Ptm decreases. As a result, the volume of the structure decreases, the pressure within increases, and as a result volume (in this case coronary blood) is translocated from this compartment to the next. Resistance to flow has increased, and flow is now proportional to the pressure gradient Pi—Ps (zone II conditions). With a greater increase in the Ps, the Ptm decreases further, and as the Ptm becomes negative, the structure collapses, Ps > Pi, and flow ceases (zone I conditions).

Throughout the cardiac cycle, ventricular pressure is transmitted to the myocardial interstitium, with myocardial tissue pressure approaching ventricular pressure in the subendocardial region and myocardial tissue pressure in the subepicardial region approaching pleural pressure [5–8]. Contributing to myocardial tissue pressure is the internal myocardial stress that is developed because of the deformation and contraction of muscle fibers [7]. With significant elevations in myocardial tissue pressure, the surrounding pressure increases, and transmural pressure decreases, resulting in the creation of zone I and II conditions.

For the LV, during systole zone I conditions are created in the subendocardium as Ps is greater than Pi and flow ceases. In the subepicardium, zone II conditions are created as Pi becomes greater than Ps, but Ps > Po. Flow is present and is proportional to Pi—Ps. If right atrial pressure rises above myocardial tissue pressure, then Pi > Po > Ps, and flow is proportional to the pressure gradient between the coronary artery and right atrium. During diastole, myocardial pressure is significantly less, zone II and III conditions exist, and flow is proportional to Pi—Ps and Pi—right atrial pressure, respectively. In contrast, because RV myocardial tissue pressure is much less than for the LV, zone II and III conditions exist throughout the myocardium and cardiac cycle, resulting in continuous flow. As a result, flow to the LV subendocardium is the most vulnerable to these compressive effects. And because perfusion of the subendocardium is limited to diastole, it is very dependent on an adequate diastolic filling period and is particularly affected by tachycardia.

Regulation of Coronary Blood Flow

The two major determinants of coronary flow are coronary arterial pressure and myocardial oxygen demand. For a given oxygen demand, coronary flow is independent of arterial perfusion pressure, which is referred to as pressure autoregulation. For a given coronary artery perfusion pressure, coronary flow changes in parallel with oxygen demand, which is referred to as metabolic autoregulation. The primary determinant of coronary blood flow and myocardial DO_2 is metabolic demand.

The tight coupling of coronary flow to myocardial oxygen demand is mediated by metabolites such as adenosine and modulated through corresponding changes in coronary vascular resistance, matching coronary flow and oxygen DO_2 with oxygen demand. With moderate increases in myocardial oxygen demand, a corresponding increase in coronary flow and myocardial DO_2 maintains the arterial-venous oxygen content difference ($AVDO_2$). With greater increases in metabolic demand, the $AVDO_2$ increases despite the significant increase in coronary blood flow and DO_2 [9].

Coronary pressure autoregulation maintains a relatively constant blood flow despite changes in the coronary perfusion pressure. Figure 4.5 illustrates this

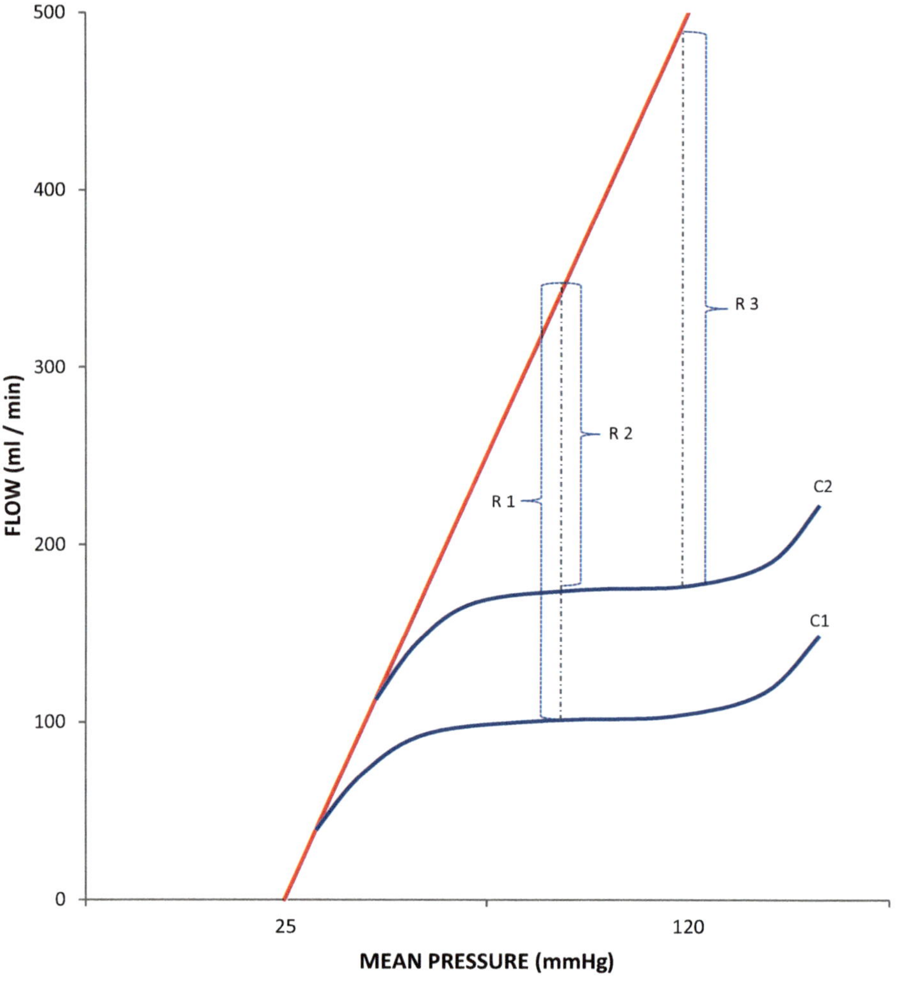

Fig. 4.5 *Coronary pressure autoregulation and coronary flow reserve.* Coronary flow is independent of coronary pressure over a wide range of pressures. Above or below the upper and lower inflection points, flow becomes pressure passive because at these pressures maximal vasoconstriction and vasodilation have occurred. C1 represents a normal LV, where C2 represents a LV that has elevated baseline flow and thus DO_2 due to either a decrease in arterial oxygen content (anemia or hypoxemia) or increase in oxygen demand. For a given coronary pressure, flow is greater for C2 than for C1. Thus, C2 has reduced coronary flow reserve (R2 < R1). With an increase in the perfusion pressure, coronary flow reserve increases (R3 > R2). Conversely, elevated LV diastolic pressure decreases coronary flow reserve for the subendocardial region

concept. This relationship between flow and pressure for a given metabolic demand (myogenic response) is also modulated through corresponding changes in coronary vascular resistance. The pressure at which resistance vessels become maximally dilated is the lowest pressure at which flow is sustained and is referred to as the lower limit of pressure autoregulation. For pressures below this lower inflection point, flow becomes pressure dependent.

Coronary flow reserve is an important concept that may be defined as the maximum increment in flow that may occur for a given perfusion pressure (Fig. 4.5) [9–11]. Coronary flow reserve is decreased when resting flow is increased, which occurs with increases in metabolic demand (increases in contractility, ventricular loading conditions, heart rate, and muscle mass) and with a decrease in arterial oxygen content (anemia or hypoxemia) [9–11]. Coronary flow reserve for the LV is also decreased when the diastolic time available for subendocardial perfusion is reduced or when the extravascular compressive effects are elevated during diastole as with elevated LV diastolic pressure.

What constitutes an adequate coronary perfusion pressure is not clear. For children, perfusion pressures are age-dependent, and there is no consensus on which approach to use for defining an adequate systemic and thus coronary perfusion pressure [11, 12]. For adults, the consensus-driven recommendations on minimum systemic arterial pressure are a mean blood pressure of >65 mmHg and a coronary perfusion pressure of >40–50 mmHg [13, 14]. For the reasons discussed, it is also important to consider alterations in myocardial oxygen demand and LV diastolic pressure.

Summary

An understanding of the determinants of myocardial VO_2 and DO_2 is essential for understanding the pathophysiological basis and management of cardiovascular disease. Consideration should be given not only to consensus-driven recommendations for minimum arterial blood pressures but also to the determinants of the pressure gradient for coronary perfusion.

References

1. Braunwald E. Myocardial oxygen consumption: the quest for its determinants and some clinical fallout. J Am Coll Cardiol. 1999;34:1365–8.
2. Suga H. Global cardiac function: mechano-energetico-informatics. J Biomech. 2003;36:713–20.
3. Suga H. Ventricular energetics. Physiol Rev. 1990;70:247–77.
4. Goodwill AG, Dick GM, Kiel AX, et al. Regulation of coronary blood flow. Compr Physiol. 2017;7:321–82.
5. Duncker DJ, Koller A, Merkus D, et al. Regulation of coronary blood flow in health and ischemic heart disease. Prog Cardiovasc Dis. 2015;57:409–22.

6. van de Hoef TP, Nolte F, Rolandi MC, et al. Coronary pressure-flow relations as basis for the understanding of coronary physiology. J Mol Cell Cardiol. 2012;52:786–93.
7. Kassab GS, Algranati D, Lanir Y. Myocardial-vessel interaction: role of LV pressure and myocardial contractility. Med Biol Eng Comput. 2013;51:729–39.
8. Duncker DJ, Bache RJ. Regulation of coronary blood flow during exercise. Physiol Rev. 2008;88:1009–86.
9. Hoffman JIE, Spaan JAE. Pressure-flow relations in coronary circulation. Physiol Rev. 1990;70:331–90.
10. Hoffman JIE. Maximal coronary flow and the concept of coronary vascular reserve. Circulation. 1984;70:153–9.
11. Weiss SL, Peters MJ, Alhazzani W, et al. Surviving sepsis campaign international guidelines for the management of septic shock and sepsis-associated organ dysfunction in children. Pediatr Crit Care Med. 2020;21:e52–e106.
12. Haque IU, Zaritsky AL. Analysis of the evidence for the lower limit of systolic and mean arterial pressure in children. Pediatr Crit Care Med. 2007;8:138–44.
13. Van Diepen S, Katz JN, Albert NM, et al. Contemporary management of cardiogenic shock. A scientific statement from the American Heart Association. Circulation. 2017;136:e232–68.
14. Levy B, Bastien O, Bendjelid K, et al. Experts' recommendations for the management of adult patients with cardiogenic shock. Ann Intensive Care. 2015;5(17):1–10.

Chapter 5
Heart-Lung Interactions

Ronald A. Bronicki and Lara S. Shekerdemian

Introduction

An understanding of the interactions between the respiratory and circulatory systems is essential for understanding the pathophysiology, assessment, and management of critical illness. In this review, we discuss the physiologic underpinnings of cardiopulmonary interactions: the volume-pressure and pressure-flow relationships applied to elastic structures in the cardiovascular and pulmonary systems; the effects of respiration and changes in intrathoracic pressure on right and left ventricular loading conditions; and the central role of these interactions in diseases commonly encountered in critical care medicine. An understanding of these complex cardiopulmonary interactions is essential to the management of critically ill patients.

Volume-Pressure and Pressure-Flow Relationships for an Elastic Structure

The extent to which an elastic structure undergoes deformation in response to a force depends on the magnitude and direction of the pressure exerted across its wall or its transmural pressure (Ptm), the difference between the inside and surrounding pressures, and its compliance, which is inversely related to elastance. A positive Ptm is a distending pressure, a negative Ptm a collapsing pressure. Compliance is a

R. A. Bronicki (✉) · L. S. Shekerdemian
Baylor College of Medicine, Texas Children's Hospital, Houston, TX, USA
e-mail: rxbronic@texaschildrens.org; lssheker@texaschildrens.org

R. A. Bronicki et al. (eds.), *Simulation in Cardiovascular Critical Care Medicine*, https://doi.org/10.1007/978-3-031-63557-1_5

measure of the distensibility of an elastic structure and is determined by the change in volume for a change in Ptm, where for a given Ptm a more compliant structure undergoes greater deformation than a less compliant structure.

An elastic structure may also be viewed in terms of its capacitance, which is the volume of fluid contained in the structure for a given Ptm and includes unstressed and stressed volumes. The amount of volume a structure can accommodate without generating a Ptm is referred to as the unstressed volume. The stressed volume is the additional volume that results in a positive Ptm.

The physical properties that govern the flow of fluids (liquid or air) through conducting passages, such as vessels and airways, whether rigid or collapsible, are based on the general laws of hydrodynamics. The behavior of flow (Q) through a collapsible structure depends on the inflow pressure (Pi), outflow pressure (Po), the surrounding pressure (Ps), the Ptm, and the compliance of the structure (Fig. 5.1). When the Ptm throughout the structure is positive, the tube is widely patent, and Q is proportional to the pressure gradient Pi—Po (also known as zone III conditions). With a constant Pi and Po, as the Ps increases, the Ptm decreases. As a result, the volume of the structure decreases, the pressure within increases, and as a result volume is translocated from this compartment to the next. Resistance to flow has increased, and flow is now proportional to the pressure gradient Pi—Ps (zone II conditions). With a greater increase in the Ps, the Ptm decreases further, and as the Ptm becomes negative, the structure collapses, Ps > Pi, and flow ceases (zone I conditions). The physiologic significance of these principles is that many structures within the pulmonary and cardiovascular systems behave analogously as intrathoracic, intra-abdominal, and intravascular pressures and volumes vary.

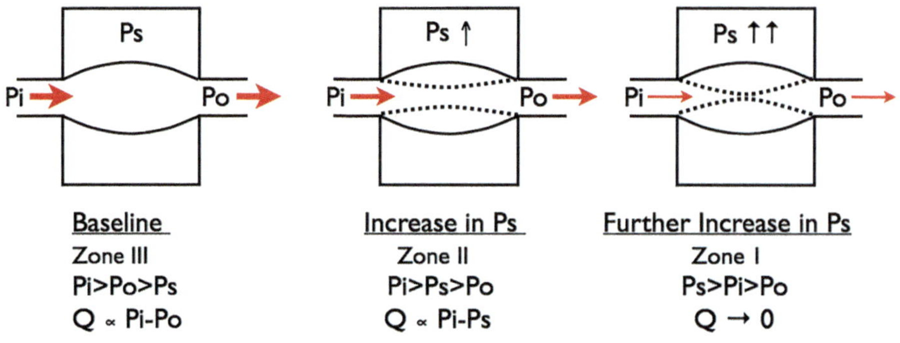

Fig. 5.1 *General principles of hydrodynamics.* Pi, Po, and Ps represent inlet, outlet, and surrounding pressure, respectively. At low Ps, the magnitude of flow through the tube is principally governed by the difference between Pi and Po (zone III conditions). If Ps is increased above Po, resistance to flow has increased and flow is governed by the difference between Pi and Ps (zone II conditions). Further increases in Ps to levels greater than Pi result in cessation of flow

The Determinants of Systemic Venous Return

The determinants of systemic venous return are a matter of controversy [1–2]. According to Guyton's theory, systemic venous return is proportional to the difference between the mean systemic pressure (Pms) and right atrial pressure and is inversely related to resistance to systemic venous return [3–6].

Resistance to systemic venous return is minimally affected by changes in arterial resistance [6]. Venous resistance is the primary determinant of resistance to systemic venous return and may be estimated as Pms—central venous pressure/cardiac output. Venous resistance remains remarkably constant despite large adrenergic stimulation [6–10]. However, resistance to systemic venous return changes appreciably with extremes in viscosity, an arteriovenous fistula, and with collapse of the vena cava due to the generation of a marked negative Ptm at the thoracic inlet (to be discussed).

The mean circulatory filling pressure (Pmcf) is the pressure that would be measured at all points in the entire circulation if the heart was arrested and blood was allowed to redistribute and the pressures to equilibrate prior to activation of compensatory circulatory reflexes [1, 3, 4–6]. The Pms is the pressure that would be measured at any given point in the systemic circulation under no flow conditions. The two pressures are equal under conditions of no flow. Each pressure is a measure of the degree of filling, which is a function of intravascular volume and vascular capacitance. As intravascular volume increases or capacitance decreases, the pressures rise. The Pmcf is determined largely by the Pms as the capacity of pulmonary circulation is low. For this reason, the Pmcf and Pms may be viewed as interchangeable. When relative functions of the right and left ventricle (RV, LV) and/or vascular resistance or capacitance are altered, Pms can be higher or lower than Pmcf.

The vast majority of vascular capacitance and thus blood volume resides with and within the systemic venous reservoirs, respectively [1, 3–5, 11–13]. These venous reservoirs, the most important of which are located within splanchnic, splenic, and hepatic circulations, are 18 times more compliant than the systemic arterial resistance vessels and thus contain most of intravascular volume (upwards of 70% of total). For these reasons, the Pms may be viewed as the pressure that is present within the venous reservoirs. Consequently, alterations in intravascular volume and venomotor tone have a profound impact on the Pms and in turn systemic venous return and play a prominent role in the pathophysiology of critical illness.

Guyton and colleagues demonstrated in normal dogs that the Pms is 7 mmHg, and the mean right atrial pressure is 2 mmHg, producing a driving pressure for systemic venous return of 5 mmHg [12, 13]. Intravascular volume expansion increases the Pms in a linear manner. Without compensatory circulatory reflexes, an increase in blood volume by 14% doubles the Pms from its normal value of 7 mmHg, whereas a decrease in blood volume of some 15% decreases the Pms to 0 mmHg. An increase in venomotor tone reduces the capacity of the venous reservoirs, increasing the pressure within and translocating volume from the reservoirs [12, 13]. Guyton and colleagues demonstrated that the removal of all vasomotor tone drops the Pms from

7 to 5 mmHg, while maximal vasomotor tone precipitated by the Cushing reflex generated a progressive increase in the Pms, which plateaued at 15 mmHg [12, 13].

Guyton's model of the circulation and the determinants of systemic venous return may be analogously compared to the flow of water into and out of a bathtub, where the tub is the venous reservoir; the tap is arterial inflow; and a drain located on the side allows for systemic venous return (Fig. 5.2) [1, 3]. The flow out of the tub is determined by the diameter of the tub opening (venous resistance), which was discussed above; the height of the column of water above the drain, which is referred to as the stressed blood volume (SBV); and over time the arterial inflow.

With a drain opening on its side, there is no drainage until the height of the water reaches the opening. The volume below this level does not contribute to the hydrostatic pressure that drives volume out of the tub and is analogous to an unstressed blood volume (UBV). The SBV creates the pressure head driving water from the tub. In the normal circulation, the UBV is roughly 4 L and the SBV 1L. The Pms is the hydrostatic pressure gradient in the tub. The Pms is 0 mmHg until the total blood volume (TBV) is upwards of 2 L, and it does exceed 2.5 mmHg until the TBV is some 4 L.

Without a change in venomotor tone, the Pms and SBV trend in parallel. With, for example, a blood transfusion or phlebotomy, SBV and Pms increase and decrease, respectively, while the UBV remains constant. Changes in venomotor tone, venoconstriction or venodilation, alter the ratio of SBV to UBV, while TBV remains constant. For example, venoconstriction decreases the UBV while increasing the SBV and Pms.

In this analogy, the pressure in the tap (systemic arterial pressure) does not affect flow coming from the tub (systemic venous return). The tap alters outflow only to the extent that the change in volume (cardiac output) flowing into the tub over time causes the height of water in the tub to change [1, 3]. Because the surface of the tub is very large compared to the height of water (i.e., highly compliant reservoirs with significant capacitance), arterial inflow has little effect on the hydrostatic pressure. If the surface area of the tub was much less relative to the height of water, the inflow would have a much greater effect on outflow as a much smaller change in volume would have a disproportionate effect on hydrostatic pressure [1, 3].

The downstream pressure opposing systemic venous return is the right atrial pressure, which is affected by several factors, including cardiac function, pericardial disease, and changes in intrathoracic pressure (ITP). During spontaneous respiration, ITP decreases, the Ptm for the right atrium increases, and as a result the right atrium distends and the pressure within falls, driving systemic venous return. Contributing to the pressure gradient for systemic venous return during spontaneous respiration is diaphragmatic descent, which increases intra-abdominal pressure, causing the Ptm and the capacity of the intra-abdominal venous reservoirs to decrease and the pressure within to rise [14–17]. This creates a longitudinal pressure gradient for systemic venous return from the largest of venous reservoirs. In other words, during inspiration, systemic venous return from the abdominal compartment results from a phasic decrease in right atrial pressure and increase in the

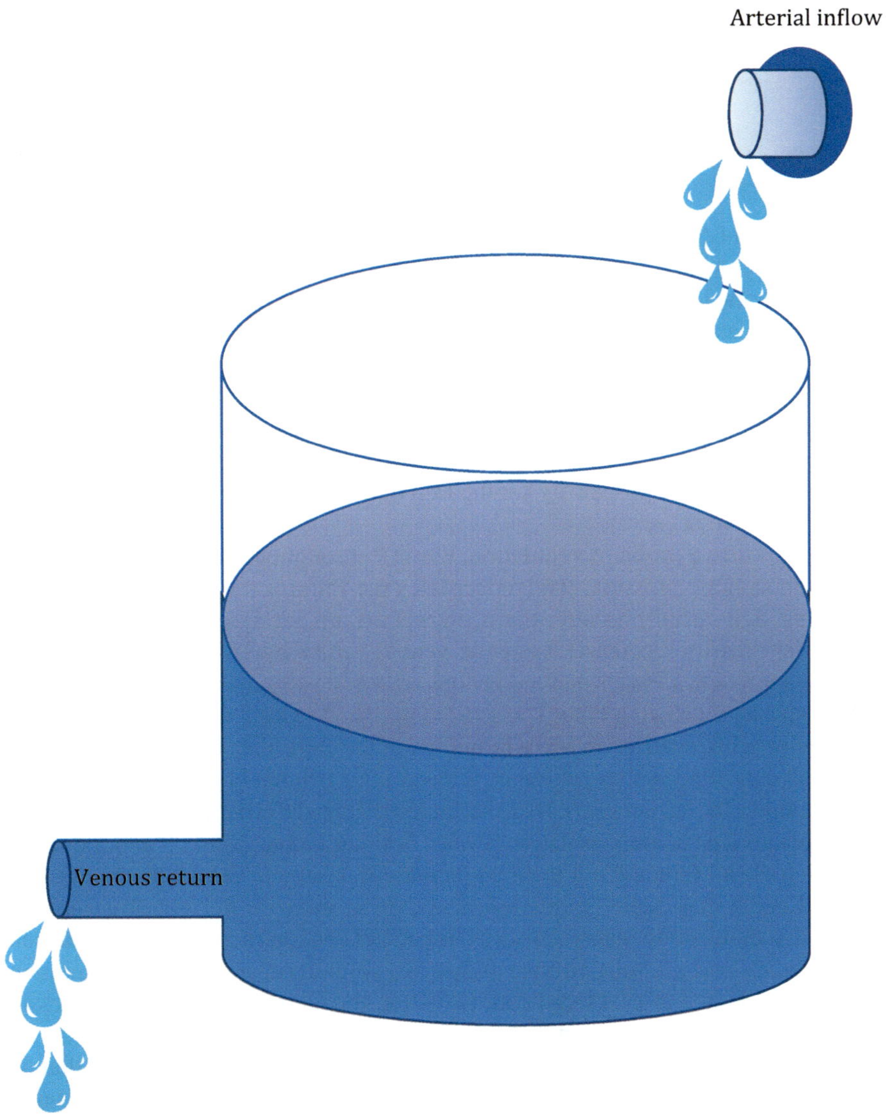

Fig. 5.2 *Systemic venous return.* Guyton's model of the circulation and the determinants of systemic venous return may be analogously compared to flow of water into and out of a bathtub, where the tub is the venous reservoir, flow from the drain is systemic venous return, resistance to systemic venous return is represented by the diameter of the drain, and the tap is arterial inflow. Flow out of the tub is determined by the height of the column of water above the drain and the diameter of the tub opening. The volume of water above the drain is referred to as the stressed blood volume (SBV), the volume below the hole is referred to as the unstressed blood volume (UBV). The height of the water above the drain increases with intravascular volume expansion, which increases total blood volume (TBV) and SBV. An increase in venomotor tone increases the SBV but does so without altering TBV. The tap (cardiac output) alters systemic venous return only to the extent that the change in volume flowing into the tub over time causes the height of water in the tub to change

Pms within the abdominal venous reservoirs, in contrast to venous return from the head and neck vessels, which are exposed to atmospheric pressure.

The Effects of Respiration on Systemic Venous Return

With exaggerated spontaneous breathing, the negative ITP is transmitted to the right atrium and vena cavae as they enter the thorax. As the vascular Ptm becomes negative at the thoracic inlet, as may occur with marked inspiratory effort, the vena cava may collapse as they enter the chest, limiting venous return (zone I conditions are created) [18]. Further decreases in right atrial pressure would have no effect on systemic venous return because flow is now a function of the difference between Pms and atmospheric pressure (for the superior vena cava) or abdominal pressure (for the inferior vena cava). When the outflow or downstream pressure is elevated, as in heart failure, the propensity for the Ptm of the vena cava at the thoracic inlet to become negative decreases.

During positive pressure ventilation, the ITP throughout the respiratory cycle is above atmospheric pressure, which decreases the Ptm for the right atrium, thereby increasing right atrial pressure. For a given Pms, an increase of only 1 mmHg in right atrial pressure decreases systemic venous return by 14%. As the right atrial pressure approaches Pms, systemic venous return ceases unless circulatory reflexes compensate by increasing Pms. This is accomplished acutely with adrenergic stimulation, with venoconstriction and a reduction in the capacitance of the venous reservoirs, and over time with retention of intravascular volume [19–22].

It is important to recognize that the increase in right atrial pressure that occurs during positive pressure ventilation results from an increase in ITP and a decrease in the right atrial Ptm and not from an increase in systemic venous return and right atrial filling. It may seem counterintuitive that an increase in right atrial pressure may be associated with a decrease in systemic venous return, right atrial filling, and ultimately RV end diastolic volume and stroke volume because right atrial pressure is used as an indicator of RV preload. However, the increase in right atrial pressure is due to a decrease in its effective compliance resulting from an increase in the surrounding pressure (Fig. 5.3) [23–27]. Pinsky and colleagues demonstrated that it is the effect of interventions such as changes in ITP or intravascular volume on the right atrial Ptm and not the right atrial pressure per se that correlates with RV preload and stroke volume [28].

In addition to the adequacy of compensatory circulatory reflexes, the extent to which systemic venous return is affected by positive pressure ventilation depends on where the RV resides on its pressure stroke volume curve. If RV end diastolic volume is normal or reduced, a decrease in systemic venous return will cause RV stroke volume to decrease. If, however, the RV resides on the flat portion of its pressure stroke volume curve, a decrease in systemic venous return will have little if any impact on stroke volume.

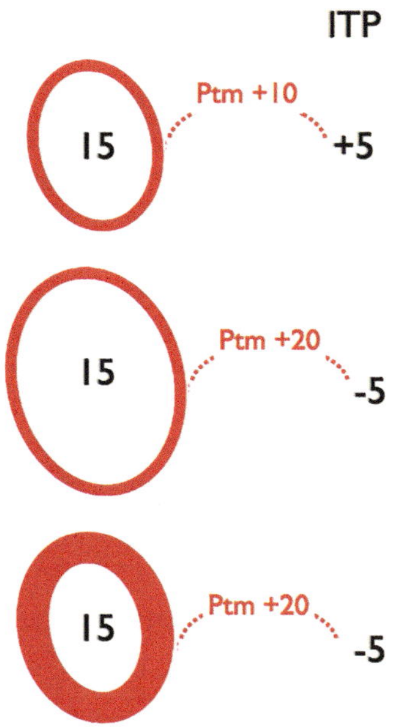

Fig. 5.3 *Alterations in the effective compliance of the heart.* The relationship of ventricular diastolic pressure (15 for each ventricle), ventricular compliance (chamber thickness), and intrathoracic pressure (ITP) to ventricular filling. The top and middle ventricles have the same diastolic pressure and compliance, but the middle chamber fills to a greater extent because its surrounding pressure (ITP) is −5, which generates a transmural pressure (Ptm) that is two-fold higher. The middle and lower ventricles have the same filling pressure and surrounding pressure, but the bottom ventricle fills less because its compliance is less

The impact of positive pressure ventilation on the circulation is also influenced by respiratory mechanics. The impact of an increase in ITP on the pressure gradient for systemic venous return depends on the magnitude of airway pressure and the degree to which lung compliance is reduced, the latter of which in part determines the extent to which airway pressure is transmitted to the cardiac fossa [25–27]. Another consideration is the impact of changes in chest wall compliance on the transmission of airway pressure to intrathoracic structures.

The respiratory system includes the lung and chest wall, and the overall mechanical behavior depends on the mechanical characteristics of its components and their interactions [29]. The chest wall, consisting of the thoracic cage and diaphragm (the latter mechanically links the abdominal cavity to the thorax), and lungs are in series and may be expressed as follows when airway resistance is minimal: Paw = Ptp + Ppl and Etot = El + Ecw, where Paw is static airway pressure, Ptp is transpulmonary pressure, Ppl is pleural pressure, Etot is total respiratory system elastance (elastance is inversely related to compliance), El is lung elastance, and Ecw is chest wall elastance [29]. Rearranging the equation to Ppl = Paw X Ecw / Etot enables us to consider the impact of changes in lung and chest wall elastance on pleural pressure or

ITP and therefore the impact of airway pressure on RV loading conditions under a variety of conditions [25, 29–31].

For a given airway pressure, increases in chest wall elastance increase ITP, decreasing the effective compliance of the right heart. For the same airway pressure, as pleural pressure rises the transpulmonary pressure decreases, decreasing end expiratory lung volume and tidal volume, with an indeterminate effect on RV afterload (decruitment and hypoxic pulmonary vasoconstriction versus decreasing the extent of alveolar overdistension and the proportion of lung regions under zone I and II conditions). Conversely, for a given airway pressure, as lung elastance increases, the transmission of airway pressure and thus pleural pressure decreases. Chest wall elastance may be elevated due to several factors, including chest wall edema and pleural effusions, as well as factors responsible for increasing abdominal pressure, such as obesity, ascites, and visceromegaly [25, 29–31].

The Effects of Respiration on Right Ventricular Afterload

Respiration affects pulmonary vascular resistance (PVR) by altering blood pH, alveolar oxygen tension, and lung volumes. Respiratory and metabolic alkalosis induces pulmonary vascular vasodilation, whereas acidosis causes vasoconstriction.

Respiration also affects PVR by altering lung volumes. This cardiopulmonary interaction is not mediated by changes in ITP per se but rather results from changes in the alveolar Ptm, regardless of the mode of ventilation, and lung compliance. Alveolar vessels lie within the septa, which separate adjacent alveoli. Alveolar pressure is the surrounding pressure for these vessels. Extra-alveolar vessels are located in the interstitium and are exposed to intrapleural pressure. Because alveolar and extra-alveolar vessels are in series, the resistance provided by each is additive. Functional residual capacity (FRC) is the lung volume from which normal tidal volume breathing occurs. PVR is lowest near the FRC and increases at both high and low lung volumes.

At low lung volumes, the radial traction provided by the pulmonary interstitium diminishes, leading to a decrease in the cross-sectional area of the extra-alveolar vessel. In addition, at low end-expiratory lung volumes, alveoli collapse and hypoxic pulmonary vasoconstriction ensues, and the resistance of extra-alveolar vessels increases further. However, the Ptm of alveolar vessels increases at low lung volumes because the alveolar Ptm falls. Nonetheless, the net effect is for PVR to increase with lung volumes well below FRC.

As lung volumes rise well above FRC, PVR increases. Large tidal volumes or tidal volumes superimposed on an elevated FRC significantly increase PVR. With large lung volumes, distended alveoli compress interalveolar vessels, decreasing the Ptm for the interalveolar vessel (creating zone I and II conditions) and increasing PVR. With positive pressure ventilation, the interstitial pressure is positive, decreasing the Ptm for the extra-alveolar vessels as well, contributing to positive pressure ventilation-induced increases in PVR. In other words, during positive pressure ventilation, alveolar and intrapleural pressures are positive during inspiration and expiration, and resistance is elevated in both alveolar and extra-alveolar vessels throughout the respiratory cycle. This contrasts with an increase in lung volume due to negative pressure ventilation where interstitial pressure is negative. This is an important consideration when using positive pressure ventilation, particularly in patients with a normal pulmonary venous pressure and in patients with underlying pulmonary vascular disease and right heart dysfunction (to be discussed below).

The extent to which lung volume affects PVR also depends on pulmonary vascular hydrostatic pressures. In the lung, pulmonary arterial pressure is the inflow pressure (Pi), pulmonary venous pressure is the outflow downstream pressure (Po), and alveolar pressure is the surrounding pressure (Ps). In addition, there is a vertical hydrostatic pressure gradient from the most dependent to the most superior portions of the lung. Because the weight of air is negligible, there is no measurable vertical gradient for alveolar pressure. In the gravity-dependent portions of the lung, Pi and Po are greater than Ps, and the Ptm for the alveolar vessel is positive throughout (zone III conditions) (Fig. 5.1). With progression to the non-gravity-dependent regions of the lung, PVR begins to increase as Ps becomes greater than Pv but remains less than Pi (zone II conditions) (Fig. 5.1). If Ps becomes greater than Pi and the Ptm for the alveolar vessel becomes negative, the vessel collapses and flow ceases (zone I conditions) (Fig. 5.1). In the absence of cardiopulmonary disease, zone I conditions do not exist. However, the proportion of lung units under zone I and II conditions increases in a variety of clinical settings. The use of positive pressure ventilation in patients with a normal Po (pulmonary venous pressure) increases the proportion of lung units under zone I and II conditions. Conversely, left heart failure with its associated pulmonary venous hypertension will increase the proportion of lung units under zone III conditions, rendering the pulmonary vasculature less vulnerable to large lung volume induced increases in PVR.

The Effects of Respiration on Left Ventricular Preload

Respiration affects LV preload by altering RV loading conditions and its effective compliance, as reviewed above. Another important determinant of the impact of respiration on LV preload is RV systolic function. As a thin-walled structure that functions as a bellow during shortening, the unprepared RV has much less contractile reserve than the LV and is therefore much more sensitive to increases in afterload [32]. Further, with positive pressure ventilation inducing increases in RV afterload, the adverse effect of increased ITP on the pressure gradient for systemic venous return may limit the extent of RV preload reserve, contributing to a fall in RV output.

Right heart dysfunction can compromise LV filling by three mechanisms. In addition to a decrease in RV stroke volume and output, right heart dysfunction compromises LV output due to ventricular interdependence (Fig. 5.4) [32]. RV dysfunction leads to RV diastolic hypertension, which decreases the normal trans-septal pressure gradient. Under normal conditions, LV diastoic pressure is greater than RV diastolic pressure casuing the interventricular septum to bow into the RV (Fig. 5.4). With RV diastolic hypertension, the interventricular septum occupies a more neutral position between the two ventricles (Fig. 5.4). If RV diastoic pressures pressure was to rise above LV diastolic pressure, the septum would bow into the LV. In either case, the LV becomes restrained not only by RV pressure and the deviated septum but also by the pericardium. These factors decrease the effective compliance of the LV (Fig. 5.3). Even though the LV filling pressure may be maintained, intrapericardial pressure has risen to a greater extent, and the net effect is a reduced LV diastolic Ptm and LV filling. This phenomenon is known as *diastolic ventricular interdependence*. This also occurs in the normal circulation albeit to a lesser extent. During spontaneous respiration, increases in systemic venous return and RV filling and pressure alter the position of the interventricular septum. This mechanism is the diastolic component of pulsus paradoxus, the decrease in systolic arterial blood pressure that occurs during spontaneous inspiration [33].

Lastly, as LV filling decreases, its ability to generate pressure is diminished. The significance of this as it relates to the circulation with RV failure due to an increased RV afterload is that the LV is responsible for generating upwards of 40% of RV systolic pressure [34]. This decrease in LV assistance to RV ejection leads to further increases in RV volume and pressure, which further impairs LV filling and pressure-generating capabilities. This phenomenon is known as *systolic ventricular interdependence* and plays an essential role in the pathophysiology of low cardiac output due to pulmonary arterial hypertension.

The overall impact of positive pressure ventilation on the right heart depends on the extent to which increases in ITP are transmitted to thoracic structures and on the extent to which changes in ITP affect right ventricular loading conditions.

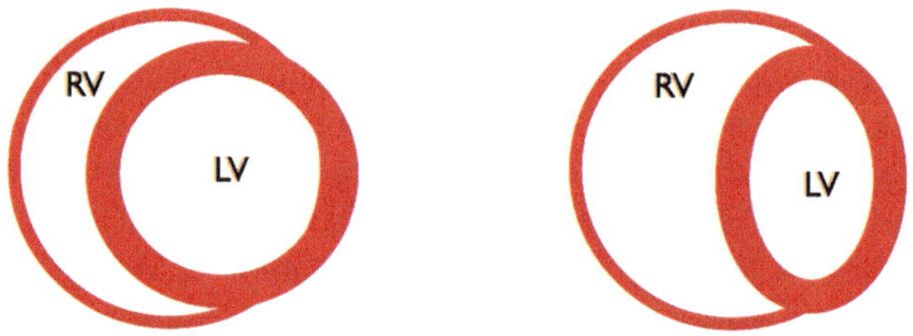

Fig. 5.4 *Ventricular interdependence.* Cartoon of a parasternal short-axis view of the left ventricle (LV) and right ventricle (RV). Under normal conditions, the interventricular septum is oriented such that in the short axis, the LV is circular. Under conditions when the pressure in the RV is elevated, the interventricular septum is displaced to the left, decreasing the effective compliance of the LV. Without an increase in the LV diastolic transmural pressure, LV filling decreases

The Effects of Respiration on Left Ventricular Afterload

Respiration has a profound impact on LV output. Changes in ITP impact not only the pressure gradient for systemic venous return but also the pressure gradient responsible for propelling blood from the thoracic cavity. While the right atrium and vena cava are much more compliant than the systemic arterial vessels, it is the compliance and Ptm for the thoracic arterial vessels that determine the extent to which changes in ITP contribute to the pressure gradient for driving blood from the chest and, therefore, to the extent that changes in ITP affect LV afterload [35–40].

During spontaneous respiration, the fall in ITP increases the Ptm and therefore the volume for the thoracic arterial system. As a result, the pressure within the thoracic arterial system decreases relative to the extrathoracic arterial system and LV afterload increases [36–40]. The effect of a decrease in ITP on LV afterload is physiological, the same as a rise in the systemic arterial blood pressure (Fig. 5.5) [35]. According to Laplace's law, LV afterload increases as the systolic Ptm increases which occurs with a decrease in ITP and rise in systemic arterial systolic pressure.

If the fall in ITP occurs during ventricular diastole, antegrade flow runoff decreases, resulting in an increase in thoracic arterial blood volume and an increase in the inertial forces opposing ejection during the following systole [36–40]. A fall in ITP during ventricular systole decreases the egress of blood from the thorax as well as LV ejection and stroke volume [36–40]. The distension of the thoracic arterial vessels and the decrease in LV output are responsible for the decrease in blood pressure during systole that occurs with spontaneous respiration and is the mechanism responsible for the systolic component of pulsus paradoxus [36–40]. As LV systolic function wanes or as ITP becomes more negative, the importance of respiration on LV afterload increases (Fig. 5.5).

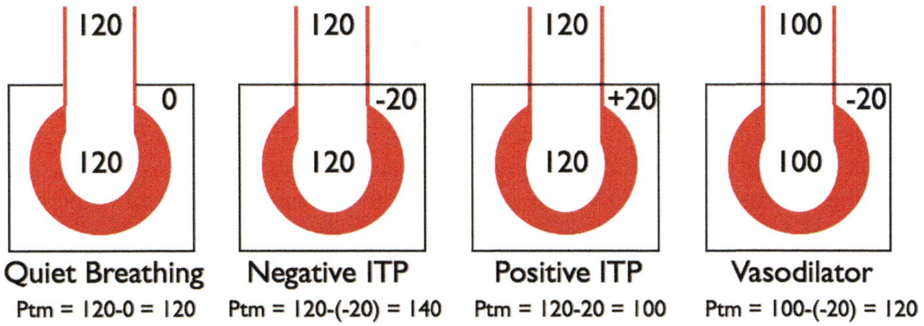

Fig. 5.5 *Impact of changes in intrathoracic pressure (ITP) on left ventricular (LV) afterload.* During periods of quiet breathing in which ITP is 0, the LV transmural pressure (Ptm) (LV afterload) is equal to LV systolic pressure (120 mm Hg) (left-hand panel). When ITP is negative (−20), the LV Ptm rises to 140 mmHg. The opposite occurs when positive pressure ventilation eliminates exaggerated negative ITP, as may be seen in cardiogenic pulmonary edema (the Ptm is reduced by nearly 30% to 100 mmHg). The LV Ptm may also be lowered pharmacologically by reducing systemic arterial resistance and aortic pressure (right-hand panel). ITP (cm H_20) has been converted to pressure in mmHg

During positive pressure ventilation, the decrease in Ptm for the thoracic arterial system increases the pressure within creating a waterfall-like effect, driving blood into the extrathoracic compartments. If the increase in ITP is confined to diastole, the LV ejects into a relatively depleted thoracic aorta with reduced inertial forces opposing ejection, while a selective increase in ITP during ventricular systole augments LV ejection without compromising the gradient for systemic venous return [36–40]. An increase in ITP therefore unloads the LV while increasing aortic diastolic and systolic pressures ("reverse pulsus paradoxus") [41]. Even though aortic pressure increases, the LV Ptm has decreased, as ITP has risen to a greater extent than LV and thoracic arterial pressures.

Understanding the physiologic principles that govern the interplay between cardiovascular and respiratory systems is essential to optimizing the care of critically ill patients. Consideration must be given to intravascular volume status and the function of the venous capacitance vessels; RV and LV diastolic and systolic function; RV and LV afterload; and the extent to which ventricular interdependence and neurohormonal activation are contributing to the pathophysiologic processes.

Cardiopulmonary Interactions in Patients with Congenital and Acquired Cardiac Disease

Left Ventricular Systolic Failure

A ventricle with impaired contractility is particularly sensitive to ventricular afterload. In patients with primarily impaired LV systolic function, stroke volume is reduced despite elevated end diastolic volume. Thus, the predominant effect of changes in ITP is on LV afterload. So long as the ventricle resides on the flat portion of its pressure stroke volume curve, an increase in ITP will cause stroke volume and cardiac output to increase [42–44]. If, however, the incremental change in ITP leads to an inadequate end diastolic volume, stroke volume and cardiac output will decrease. In addition, LV systolic heart failure can lead to cardiogenic pulmonary edema, which in turn results in exaggerated negative pressure breathing. This results in further neurohormonal activation, which leads to venoconstriction and an increase in SBV, and further increases in systemic vascular resistance, arterial blood pressure, and LV afterload. The heart becomes more congested, and a positive feedback cycle ensues (Fig. 5.5) [45–49]. Positive airway pressure reduces or eliminates the exaggerated decrease in ITP, decreasing sympathetic nervous system activation and improving LV loading conditions.

In addition to improving cardiac output and systemic oxygen delivery, mechanical ventilation improves the myocardial and respiratory pump oxygen supply demand relationship by reducing oxygen demand. In accordance with Laplace's principle, by decreasing LV end diastolic volume and systolic Ptm, myocardial oxygen consumption is reduced. In addition, by unloading the respiratory muscles, mechanical ventilation reduces respiratory muscle oxygen demand and in doing so allows for a redistribution of a limited cardiac output to other vital organs.

Under normal conditions, the diaphragm consumes less than 3% of global oxygen consumption and receives less than 5% of cardiac output [50]. However, with an increase in respiratory load, diaphragmatic oxygen consumption may increase to values over 50% of total oxygen consumption [50, 51]. The increase in respiratory muscle oxygen consumption correlates with an increase in minute ventilation and increases further with impairment of respiratory mechanics. Because the baseline arteriovenous oxygen content difference for the diaphragm is high, diaphragmatic blood flow must increase to meet the increase in oxygen demand, which if cardiac output is limited occurs at the expense of other vital organs [50–53]. Animal models of cardiogenic and septic shock have evaluated the distribution of cardiac output during spontaneous and mechanical ventilation [52, 53]. Viires and colleagues as well as Hussain and colleagues demonstrated that respiratory muscle blood flow increases significantly in animal models of shock [52, 53]. Both studies demonstrated that in animals receiving mechanical ventilation, respiratory muscle blood flow is significantly less and that perfusion to other vital organs, including the brain, is significantly greater than that seen in the spontaneously breathing animals.

These studies demonstrate that diaphragmatic blood flow is protected to an equal or even greater extent than is cerebral blood flow when cardiac output is limited and that by unloading the respiratory pump mechanical ventilation allows for a redistribution of a limited cardiac output to other vital organs. The importance of these principles has been demonstrated in several studies and in different lines of investigation. Rasanen and colleagues found that progressing from positive pressure ventilation to spontaneous respiration adversely affected the myocardial oxygen supply demand relationship in patients with acute myocardial infarction complicated by respiratory failure, resulting in myocardial ischemia and significant elevations in LV filling pressure [54]. Scharf and colleagues demonstrated acute LV regional akinesis in patients with preexisting LV dysfunction during performance of the Mueller maneuver (generates exaggerated negative ITP by inspiring against a closed glottis) [55]. Jubran and colleagues demonstrated in adult patients with underlying cardiopulmonary disease receiving positive pressure ventilation that patients who failed a spontaneous breathing trial were unable to increase their cardiac output to meet the metabolic demand of the respiratory muscles. This was reflected in the progressive increase in their oxygen extraction ratios and a 2.5-fold increase in LV filling pressure. In contrast those patients who tolerated the spontaneous breathing trial demonstrated a significant compensatory increase in cardiac output and maintained a normal oxygen extraction ratio and LV filling pressure [56].

In adult patients with decompensated LV systolic heart failure and pulmonary edema, meta-analyses have shown a significant reduction in the need for intubation and early mortality with noninvasive positive airway pressure [57, 58]. The long-term benefits of noninvasive positive airway pressure have also been demonstrated in adult patients with chronic LV heart failure. Haruki and colleagues found that the prolonged use of noninvasive positive pressure ventilation delivered for at least four hours per day for six months led to ventricular remodeling and significantly improved LV diastolic and systolic function [59].

Ventricular Diastolic Dysfunction

In patients with diastolic ventricular dysfunction, such as restrictive and hypertrophic cardiomyopathies and heart failure with preserved ejection fraction, LV systolic function is most often adequate if not normal. However, ventricular end diastolic volume may be reduced, and if so, one would expect the predominant effect of an increase in ITP to be on the right heart and that the determinants of the Pms would be of particular importance in these patients [60]. In hypertrophic cardiomyopathies, if the substrate for an obstruction to LV outflow is present, by decreasing LV preload and afterload, positive pressure ventilation may create or exacerbate the obstruction during systole [61].

The impact of respiration on ventricular loading conditions in the setting of ventricular diastolic disease is exemplified in the postoperative management of patients following the repair of tetralogy of Fallot. In these patients, biventricular systolic function is normal; however, RV diastolic dysfunction is common, and in a subset of these patients, restrictive RV physiology is present [62, 63]. Shekerdemian and colleagues demonstrated a significant increase in stroke volume and cardiac output when patients were converted from positive to negative pressure ventilation using a cuirass [64].

Following the Fontan procedure, as in the normal circulation, the Pms is the upstream pressure for driving systemic venous return, while the pressure within the confluence of the vena cavae and pulmonary artery is the downstream pressure [65–67]. However, because the Fontan circulation lacks a subpulmonic pumping chamber, the Pms is not only the upstream pressure for driving systemic venous return to the central confluence of the vena cavae and pulmonary artery but also the pressure responsible for driving blood across the pulmonary circulation to the common atrium [65–67]. For these reasons, the Fontan circulation is particularly sensitive to changes in ITP and impaired ventricular diastolic function, which is invariably present to varying degrees immediately following and remote from the time of surgery [68–72]. Shekerdemian and colleagues demonstrated a marked increase in pulmonary blood flow, stroke volume, and cardiac output when patients were transitioned form positive pressure to negative pressure ventilation using a cuirass immediately following and remote from the Fontan procedure [73]. Although negative pressure ventilation is impractical, the discussion highlights the impact of changes in ITP on cardiac output in the setting of diastolic dysfunction.

Cardiopulmonary Interactions in Hypoxic Respiratory Failure

Despite the use of lung-protective ventilation strategies for acute respiratory distress syndrome (ARDS), positive pressure ventilation may induce significant heart-lung interactions that adversely impact gas exchange, RV loading conditions, cardiac output, and ultimately systemic oxygen delivery [74]. More than 60% of adult patients with ARDS experience hemodynamic failure, necessitating vasoactive support [75, 76]. ARDS is frequently associated with RV dysfunction, the most severe form of which is acute cor pulmonale, which occurs in 25–30% of adult patients with ARDS [77, 78]. Further, RV dysfunction has been shown to be independently associated with a higher risk of death in these patients [79, 80]. Similar findings have been demonstrated in children with ARDS [81, 82].

As discussed, increases in ITP may compromise systemic venous return as well as the effective compliance of the RV. Additional important considerations are the effects of positive pressure ventilation on the right heart resulting from changes in alveolar Ptm, lung volume, and PVR. Jardin and colleagues evaluated patients receiving positive pressure ventilation for ARDS and found a significant decrease in RV shortening and increase in RV systolic dimensions consistent with an increase in RV afterload, which was temporally related to the inspiratory phase of positive pressure ventilation [83, 84]. RV end diastolic dimensions remained unchanged consistent with a limitation of systemic venous return since an increase in RV afterload should lead to an increase in RV end diastolic volume. Additional factors that dictate the extent to which positive pressure ventilation impacts RV output are intravascular volume status and RV systolic and diastolic function, each of which may be affected by the underlying disease process (e.g., sepsis) [85, 86].

In patients with hypoxic respiratory failure, it is important not only to consider the impact of positive airway pressure on oxygenation but also to consider its impact on cardiac output and ultimately systemic oxygen delivery.

Cardiopulmonary Interactions in Sepsis

Severe sepsis may affect virtually every aspect of respiratory and circulatory systems, compromising the function of each and setting into motion any number of heart-lung interactions [86, 87]. In addition to precipitating acute lung injury/ARDS, sepsis may impact the function of the arterial resistance and venous capacitance vessels and diastolic and systolic function of either or both ventricles. This topic is covered in Chap. 10.

Conclusion

Under normal conditions, the interplay between the respiratory and cardiovascular systems is inconsequential. However, in the presence of underlying cardiopulmonary disease, the importance of the interaction between these two organ systems cannot be overstated. A comprehensive understanding of these interactions is essential to the practice of cardiac critical care and for optimizing patient care.

References

1. Magder S. Point: counterpoint: the classical Guyton view that mean systemic pressure, right atrial pressure, and venous resistance govern venous return is/is not correct. J Appl Physiol. 2006;101:1523–5.
2. Brengelmann GL. A critical analysis of the view that right atrial pressure determines venous return. J Appl Physiol. 2003;94:849–59.
3. Magder S. Volume and its relationship to cardiac output and venous return. Crit Care. 2016;20:271.
4. Guyton AC, Jones CE, Coleman TG. Peripheral vascular contribution to cardiac output regulation—the concept of "venous return.". In: Guyton AC, Jones CE, Coleman TG, editors. Circulatory physiology: cardiac output and its regulation. 2nd ed. Philadelphia: WB Saunders; 1973. p. 173–87.
5. Rothe CF. Mean circulatory filling pressure: its meaning and measurement. J Appl Physiol. 1993;74:499–509.
6. Guyton AC, Abernathy B, Langston JB, et al. Relative importance of venous and arterial resistances in controlling venous return and cardiac output. Am J Phys. 1959;196:1008–14.
7. Guyton AC, Lindsey AW, Abernathy B, et al. Mechanism of the increased venous return and cardiac output caused by epinephrine. Am J Phys. 1958;192:126–30.
8. Hatanakah T, Potts JT. Invariance of the resistance to venous return to carotid sinus baroreflex control. Am J Phys. 1996;271(3 Pt 2):H1022–30.
9. Caldini P, Permutt S, Waddell JA, et al. Effect of epinephrine on pressure, flow, and volume relationships in the systemic circulation in dogs. Circ Res. 1974;34:606–23.
10. Greene AS, Shoukas AA. Changes in canine cardiac function and venous return curves by the carotid baroreflex. Am J Phys. 1986;251:H288–96.
11. Drees JA, Rothe CF. Reflex venoconstriction and capacity vessel pressure-volume relationships in dogs. Circ Res. 1974;34:360–73.
12. Guyton AC, Polizo D, Armstrong GG. Mean circulatory filling pressure measured immediately after cessation of heart pumping. Am J Phys. 1954;179:261–7.
13. Richardson TQ, Stallings JO, Guyton AC. Pressure-volume curves in live, intact dogs. Am J Phys. 1961;201:471–4.
14. Takata M, Wise RA, Robotham JL. Effects of abdominal pressure on venous return: abdominal vascular zone conditions. J Appl Physiol. 1990;69:1961–72.
15. Takata M, Robotham JL. Effects of inspiratory diaphragmatic descent on inferior vena caval venous return. J Appl Physiol. 1992;72:597–607.
16. Lloyd TC Jr. Effect of inspiration on inferior vena caval blood flow in dogs. J Appl Physiol. 1983;55:1701–8.
17. Karim F, Hainsworth R. Responses of abdominal vascular capacitance to stimulation of splanchnic nerves. Am J Phys. 1976;231:434–40.
18. Guyton AC, Adkins LH. Quantitative aspects of the collapse factor in relation to venous return. Am J Phys. 1954;177:523–7.

19. Fessler HE, Brower RG, Wise RA, et al. Effects of positive end-expiratory pressure on the gradient for venous return. Am Rev Respir Dis. 1991;143:19–24.
20. Payen DM, Brun-Buisson CJL, Carli PA, et al. Hemodynamic, gas exchange, and hormonal consequences of LBPP during PEEP ventilation. J Appl Physiol. 1987;62:61–70.
21. Bark H, LeRoith D, Myska M, et al. Elevations in plasma ADH levels during PEEP ventilation in the dog: mechanisms involved. Am J Phys. 1980;239:E474–80.
22. Scharf SM, Ingram RH Jr. Influence of abdominal pressure and sympathetic vasoconstriction on the cardiovascular response to positive end-expiratory pressure. Am Rev Respir Dis. 1977;116:661–70.
23. O'Quin R, Marini JJ. Pulmonary artery occlusion pressure: clinical physiology, measurement, and interpretation. Am Rev Respir Dis. 1983;128:319–26.
24. Takata M, Robotham JL. Ventricular external constraint by the lung and pericardium during positive end-expiratory pressure. Am Rev Respir Dis. 1991;143:872–5.
25. O'Quin RJ, Marini JJ, Culver BH, et al. Transmission of airway pressure to pleural space during lung edema and chest wall restriction. J Appl Physiol. 1985;59:1171–7.
26. Novak R, Matuschak GM, Pinsky MR. Effect of positive pressure ventilatory frequency on regional pleural pressure. J Appl Physiol. 1988;65:1314–23.
27. Cabrera MR, Nakamura GE, Montague DA, et al. Effect of airway pressure on pericardial pressure. Am Rev Respir Dis. 1986;140:559–67.
28. Pinsky M. Determinants of pulmonary arterial flow variation during respiration. J Appl Physiol. 1984;56:1237–45.
29. Gattinoni L, Chiumello D, Carlesso E, et al. Bench-to-bedside review: chest wall elastance in acute lung injury/acute respiratory distress syndrome patients. Crit Care. 2004;8:350–5.
30. Ranieri VM, Brienza N, Santostasi S, et al. Impairment of lung and chest wall mechanics in patients with acute respiratory distress syndrome. Role of abdominal distension. Am J Respir Crit Care Med. 1997;156:1082–91.
31. Gattinoni L, Pelosi P, Suter PM, et al. Acute respiratory distress syndrome caused by pulmonary and extrapulmonary disease. Am J Respir Crit Care Med. 1998;158:3–11.
32. Bronicki RA, Baden HP. Pathophysiology of right ventricular failure in pulmonary hypertension. Pediatr Crit Care Med. 2010;11(Suppl):S15–22.
33. Peters J, Kindred MK, Robotham JL. Transient analysis of cardiopulmonary interactions. I. Diastolic events. J Appl Physiol. 1988;64:1506–17.
34. Santamore WP, Gray L. Significant left ventricular contributions to right ventricular systolic function. Chest. 1995;107:1134–45.
35. Bronicki RA, Anas NG. Cardiopulmonary interaction. Pediatr Crit Care Med. 2009;10:313–22.
36. Fewell JE, Abendschein DR, Carlson J, et al. Mechanism of decreased right and left ventricular end-diastolic volumes during continuous positive-pressure ventilation in dogs. Circ Res. 1980;47:467–72.
37. Fessler HE, Brower RG, Wise RA, et al. Mechanism of reduced LV afterload by systolic and diastolic positive pleural pressure. J Appl Physiol. 1988;65:1244–50.
38. Peters J, Kindred MK, Robotham JL. Transient analysis of cardiopulmonary interaction. II. Systolic events. J Appl Physiol. 1988;64:1518–26.
39. Pinsky MR, Matuschak GM, Bernardi L, et al. Hemodynamic effects of cardiac cycle-specific increases in intrathoracic pressure. J Appl Physiol. 1986;60:604–12.
40. Pinsky MR, Marquez J, Martin D, et al. Ventricular assist by cardiac cycle-specific increases in intrathoracic pressure. Chest. 1987;91:709–15.
41. Massumi RA, Mason DT, Vera Z, et al. Reversed pulsus paradoxus. N Engl J Med. 1973;289:1272–5.
42. Genovese J, Moskowitz M, Tarasiuk A, et al. Effects of continuous positive airway pressure on cardiac output in normal and hypervolemic unanesthetized pigs. Am J Respir Crit Care Med. 1994;150:752–8.
43. Grace MP, Greenbaum DM. Cardiac performance in response to PEEP in patients with cardiac dysfunction. Crit Care Med. 1982;10:358–60.

44. Bradley TD, Holloway RM, McLaughlin PR, et al. Cardiac output response to continuous positive airway pressure in congestive heart failure. Am Rev Respir Dis. 1992;145:377–82.
45. Kennedy SK, Weintraub RM, Skillman JJ. Cardiorespiratory and sympathoadrenal responses during weaning from controlled ventilation. Surgery. 1977;82:233–40.
46. Somers VK, Dyken ME, Skinner JL. Autonomic and hemodynamic responses and interactions during the Mueller maneuver in humans. J Auton Nerv Syst. 1993;44:253–9.
47. Oh TE, Bhatt S, Lin ES, et al. Plasma catecholamines and oxygen consumption during weaning from mechanical ventilation. Intensive Care Med. 1991;17:199–203.
48. Morgan BJ, Denahan T, Ebert TJ. Neurocirculatory consequences of negative intrathoracic pressure vs. asphyxia during voluntary apnea. J Appl Physiol. 1993;74:2969–75.
49. Katragadda S, Xie A, Puleo D, et al. Neural mechanism of the pressor response to obstructive and nonobstructive apnea. J Appl Physiol. 1997;83:2048–54.
50. Roussos C, Macklem PT. The respiratory muscles. N Engl J Med. 1982;307:786–97.
51. Rochester DF, Bettini G. Diaphragmatic blood flow and energy expenditure in the dog. Effects of inspiratory airflow resistance and hypercapnia. J Clin Invest. 1976;57:661–72.
52. Viires N, Aubier SM, Rassidakis A, et al. Regional blood flow distribution in dog during induced hypotension and low cardiac output. J Clin Invest. 1983;72:935–47.
53. Hussain SNA, Roussos C. Distribution of respiratory muscle and organ blood flow during endotoxic shock in dogs. J Appl Physiol. 1985;59:1802–8.
54. Rasanen J, Nikki P, Heikkila J. Acute myocardial infarction complicated by respiratory failure. Chest. 1984;85:21–8.
55. Scharf SM, Bianco JA, Tow DE, et al. The effects of large negative intrathoracic pressure on left ventricular function in patients with coronary artery disease. Circulation. 1981;63:871–5.
56. Jubran A, Mathru M, Dries D, et al. Continuous recordings of mixed venous oxygen saturation during weaning from mechanical ventilation and the ramifications thereof. Am J Respir Crit Care Med. 1998;158:1763–9.
57. Winck J, Azevedo LF, Costa-Pereira A, et al. Efficacy and safety of non-invasive ventilation in the treatment of acute cardiogenic pulmonary edema—a systematic review and meta-analysis. Crit Care. 2006;10:1–18.
58. Massip J, Roque M, Sanchez B, et al. Noninvasive ventilation in acute cardiogenic pulmonary edema. JAMA. 2005;294:3124–30.
59. Haruki N, Takeuchi M, Kaku K, et al. Comparison of acute and chronic impact of adaptive servo-ventilation on left chamber geometry and function in patients with chronic heart failure. Eur J Heart Fail. 2011;10:1140–6.
60. Thomson HL, Morris-Thurgood J, Atherton J, et al. Reflex responses of venous capacitance vessels in patients with hypertrophic cardiomyopathy. Clin Sci. 1998;94:339–46.
61. Braunwald E, Oldham H Jr, Ross J, et al. The circulatory response of patients with idiopathic hypertrophic subaortic stenosis to nitroglycerin and to the Valsalva maneuver. Circulation. 1964;29:422–31.
62. Appleton CP, Hatle LK, Popp RL. Demonstration of restrictive ventricular physiology by Doppler echocardiography. J Am Coll Cardiol. 1988;11:757–68.
63. Cullen S, Shore D, Redington A. Characterization of right ventricular diastolic performance after complete repair of tetralogy of Fallot. Circulation. 1995;91:1782–9.
64. Shekerdemian LS, Bush A, Shore DF, et al. Cardiorespiratory responses to negative pressure ventilation after tetralogy of Fallot repair: a hemodynamic tool for patients with a low-output state. J Am Coll Cardiol. 1999;33:549–55.
65. Mace L, Dervanian P, Bourriez A, et al. Changes in venous return parameters associated with univentricular Fontan circulations. Am J Physiol Heart Circ Physiol. 2000;279:H2335–43.
66. Krishnan US, Taneja I, Gewitz M, et al. Peripheral vascular adaptation and orthostatic tolerance in Fontan physiology. Circulation. 2009;120:1775–83.
67. Myers CD, Ballman K, Riegle LE, et al. Mechanisms of systemic adaptation to univentricular Fontan conversion. J Thorac Cardiovasc Surg. 2010;140:850–6.

68. Williams DB, Kiernan PD, Metke MP, et al. Hemodynamic response to positive end-expiratory pressure following right atrium-pulmonary artery bypass (Fontan procedure). J Thorac Cardiovasc Surg. 1984;87:856–61.
69. Senzaki H, Masutani S, Ishido H, et al. Cardiac rest and reserve function in patients with Fontan circulation. J Am Coll Cardiol. 2006;47:2528–35.
70. Liang F, Senzaki H, Kurishima C, et al. Hemodynamic performance of the Fontan circulation compared with a normal biventricular circulation: a computational model study. Am J Physiol Heart Circ Physiol. 2014;307:H1056–72.
71. Kelley JR, Mack GW, Fahey JT. Diminished venous vascular capacitance in patients with univentricular hearts after the Fontan operation. Am J Cardiol. 1995;76:158–63.
72. Penny DJ, Rigby ML, Redington AN. Abnormal patterns of intraventricular flow and diastolic filling after the Fontan operation: evidence for incoordinate ventricular wall motion. Br Heart J. 1991;66:375–8.
73. Shekerdemian LS, Bush A, Shore DF, et al. Cardiopulmonary interactions after the Fontan operation. Augmentation of cardiac output using negative pressure ventilation. Circulation. 1997;96:3934–42.
74. Vieillard-Baron A, Matthay M, Teboul JL, et al. Experts' opinion on management of hemodynamics in ARDS patients: focus on the effects of mechanical ventilation. Intensive Care Med. 2016;42:739–49.
75. Dessap AM, Boissier F, Charron C, et al. Acute cor pulmonale during protective ventilation for acute respiratory distress syndrome: prevalence predictors, and clinical impact. Intensive Care Med. 2016;42:862–70.
76. McAuley DF, Laffey JG, O'Kane CM, et al. Simvastatin in the acute respiratory distress syndrome. N Engl J Med. 2014;371:1695–703.
77. Vieillard-Baron A, Schmitt JM, Augarde R, et al. Acute cor pulmonale in acute respiratory distress syndrome submitted to protective ventilation: incidence, clinical implications, and prognosis. Crit Care Med. 2001;29(8):1551–5.
78. Osman D, Monnet X, Castelain V, et al. Incidence and prognostic value of right ventricular failure in acute respiratory distress syndrome. Intensive Care Med. 2009;35(1):69–76.
79. Monchi M, Bellenfant F, Cariou A, et al. Early predictive factors of survival in the acute respiratory distress syndrome. A multivariate analysis. Am J Respir Crit Care Med. 1998;158:1076–81.
80. Boissier F, Katsahian S, Razazi K, et al. Prevalence and prognosis of cor pulmonale during protective ventilation for acute respiratory distress syndrome. Intensive Care Med. 2013;39:1725–33.
81. Himebauch AS, Yehya N, Wang Y, et al. New or persistent right ventricular systolic dysfunction is associated with worse outcomes in pediatric acute respiratory distress syndrome. Pediatr Crit Care Med. 2020;21:e121–8.
82. Himebauch AS, Yehya N, Wang Y, et al. Early right ventricular systolic dysfunction and pulmonary hypertension are associated with worse outcomes in pediatric acute respiratory distress syndrome. Crit Care Med. 2018;46:e1055–62.
83. Vieillard-Baron A, Loubieres Y, Schmitt J-M, et al. Cyclic changes in right ventricular output impedance during mechanical ventilation. J Appl Physiol. 1999;87:1644–50.
84. Jardin F, Viellard-Baron A. Right ventricular function and positive pressure ventilation in clinical practice: from hemodynamic subsets to respirator settings. Intensive Care Med. 2003;29:1426–34.
85. Fougeres E, Teboul J-L, Richard C, et al. Hemodynamic impact of a positive end-expiratory pressure setting in acute respiratory distress syndrome: importance of the volume status. Crit Care Med. 2010;38:802–7.
86. Funk DJ, Jacobsohn E, Kumar A. The role of venous return in critical illness and shock—part I: physiology. Crit Care Med. 2013;41:255–62.
87. Beesley SJ, Weber G, Sarge T, et al. Septic cardiomyopathy. Crit Care Med. 2018;46:625–34.

Chapter 6
Vasoactive Agents

Joseph Philip, Javier J. Lasa, and Ronald A. Bronicki

Introduction

In this review, we discuss vasoactive agents used to acutely modify cardiac and vascular function. Consideration should be given to the impact of the agent on and the underlying function of the systemic venous capacitance and the arterial resistance vessels (pulmonary and systemic circulations); right and left ventricles (lusitropy and contractility); and heart rate, including the impact of changes in heart rate on ventricular loading conditions, cardiac output, and the determinants of myocardial energetics (the myocardial oxygen supply and demand relationship).

With the application of the time-varying elastance principles (reviewed in Chap. 2), one can predict the impact of therapeutic interventions on clinical parameters used by the clinician at the bedside. With this approach, the emphasis is on the effects of each agent on the circulation rather than on the agent or class of agent selected. Differences among agents are primarily based on mechanisms of action and hemodynamic effects, and the selection of an agent is based on the patient's hemodynamic phenotype and which drug best addresses the physiological abnormalities and the objectives of therapy. This strategy avoids a formulaic approach to

J. Philip
University of Florida College of Medicine, University of Florida Health Shands Hospital, Gainesville, FL, USA
e-mail: subijo9@ufl.edu

J. J. Lasa
University of Texas Southwestern Medical School, Children's Medical Center of Dallas, Dallas, TX, USA
e-mail: javier.lasa@utsouthwestern.edu

R. A. Bronicki (✉)
Baylor College of Medicine, Texas Children's Hospital, Houston, TX, USA
e-mail: rxbronic@texaschildrens.org

R. A. Bronicki et al. (eds.), *Simulation in Cardiovascular Critical Care Medicine*, https://doi.org/10.1007/978-3-031-63557-1_6

treating diseases and enables the clinician to tailor therapies according to each patient's unique pathophysiologic state.

Catecholamines

The hemodynamic effects of catecholamines are dose-dependent and are mediated by a variety of adrenergic receptors that use the cyclic adenosine monophosphate (cAMP)-dependent signaling cascade. As intracellular cAMP increases, intracellular calcium metabolism and cellular function are altered. β_2 and $\alpha_1$adrenergic receptors are situated on vascular smooth muscle cells where they mediate vasodilation and vasoconstriction, respectively. β_1 receptors are located on cardiomyocytes where they mediate enhanced contractility and, to a lesser extent, increased heart rate. β-Adrenergic receptors experience β-agonist-mediated receptor downregulation and desensitization in which an attenuated physiologic response to β-agonists occurs with prolonged exposure to elevated levels of endogenous and exogenous catecholamines [1]. For example, in chronic heart failure, circulating and myocardial norepinephrine and epinephrine levels are chronically elevated, which leads to adrenergic receptor desensitization and a waning of the physiologic response to adrenergic agonist [2, 3]. Catecholamines are primarily metabolized by enzyme systems and have a very short half-life of less than 5 minutes, allowing for rapid titration. Catecholamines increase myocardial oxygen demand because of their chronotropic and inotropic effects.

Dopamine is the immediate precursor of norepinephrine in the endogenous catecholamine biosynthesis pathway. Approximately half of the dopamine-induced response results from dopamine-induced release of norepinephrine from sympathetic nerve terminals. Dopamine directly stimulates α, β, and dopaminergic receptors.

Dopamine in low doses (<3–5 mcg/kg/min) increases contractility and heart rate [4–9]. At higher doses (>5–10 mcg/kg/min), α-adrenergic effects predominate, resulting in vasoconstriction of venous capacitance and systemic arterial resistance vessels, with little effect on pulmonary vascular resistance [4–15].

Dobutamine is a synthetic catecholamine with an affinity for β_1 than β_2 receptors, increasing contractility and heart rate and to a lesser degree inducing vasodilation of systemic and pulmonary arterial resistance and venous capacitance vessels [5, 6, 10–16].

Epinephrine is an endogenous catecholamine that functions as a hormone. It is formed from norepinephrine through N-methylation and released by the adrenal medulla. Epinephrine increases contractility and heart rate. Additionally, in low doses (<0.1 mcg/kg/min), epinephrine reduces systemic vascular resistance, primarily due to stimulation of β_2 receptors in skeletal muscle [17–23]. This finding has also been demonstrated in patients with elevated endogenous catecholamine levels [23]. At much higher doses (>0.4–0.5 mcg/kg/min), systemic vascular resistance begins to increase with stimulation of α_1 receptors predominating [24]. While epinephrine stimulates β_2 receptors, it appears to induce venoconstriction and a reduction in venous capacitance [10–12]. The impact of epinephrine on pulmonary arterial resistance is less clear, but it appears to have little effect at low to moderate doses [13–15].

Norepinephrine is the endogenous neurotransmitter of the sympathetic nervous system. It is primarily released from terminal nerve endings and acts locally but is also secreted to a lesser extent by the adrenal medulla. Norepinephrine is a potent α_1 agonist with less affinity for β_1 receptors. As a result, norepinephrine increases peripheral arterial resistance to a greater extent than contractility. Vasoconstriction of venous capacitance decreases venous capacitance, increasing the stressed circulating blood volume [10–12]. The impact of norepinephrine on pulmonary arterial resistance is less clear, but it appears to have a limited effect [13–15].

Phenylephrine is an α-agonist that causes vasoconstriction of pulmonary and systemic arterial resistance and venous capacitance vessels [10–15, 24]. Phenylephrine has no significant β-effects.

Isoproterenol is a synthetic catecholamine that stimulates β_1 and β_2 receptors, increasing contractility and heart rate. Isoproterenol significantly vasodilates arterial resistance and venous capacitance vessels [10–16].

Milrinone

Milrinone does not act via adrenergic receptors, but rather through selective inhibition of phosphodiesterase III. As a result, milrinone is immune to the effects of chronically elevated endogenous catecholamines and adrenergic receptor desensitization, as is seen in longstanding heart failure. Phosphodiesterase inhibition leads to a reduction of cAMP degradation and subsequent increases in intracellular calcium, leading to increases in contractility as well as vasodilation of venous capacitance and pulmonary and systemic arterial resistance vessels [25]. Phosphodiesterase inhibitors are also considered the least chronotropic and arrhythmogenic of all inotropic agents. Milrinone has a relatively long half-life of 2–3 hours with notable age-dependent pharmacokinetics, making it less titratable. Milrinone is predominantly cleared via renal excretion; therefore, dosing may need to be adjusted in patients with renal insufficiency [26–28].

Nitroprusside

Nitroprusside spontaneously releases nitric oxide, which activates the soluble form of guanylate cyclase producing increased levels of cyclic guanosine monophosphate (cGMP) [29]. Nitroprusside causes dose-dependent dilation of systemic and pulmonary arterial resistance and venous capacitance vessels [29]. Nitroprusside decomposes nonenzymatically in the blood, releasing cyanide, which undergoes transsulfuration to form thiocyanate. Nitroprusside has a short half-life of two minutes; however, thiocyanate is excreted by the kidneys and has a half-life of 3 days in patients with normal renal function. While thiocyanate is not vasoactive, it does accumulate in the setting of renal failure and may cause neurotoxicity. When thiosulfate stores are depleted, cyanide toxicity ensues. Simultaneous infusion of thiosulfate with nitroprusside provides the sulfur donor necessary to prevent cyanide accumulation.

Nitroglycerin

Nitroglycerin undergoes biotransformation to yield nitric oxide. Nitroglycerin produces dose-dependent dilation of systemic and pulmonary arterial and venous capacitance vessels [30–32]. In low to moderate doses (<3 mcg/kg/minute), nitroglycerin primarily vasodilates venous capacitance vessels, while in higher doses it also vasodilates systemic arterial resistance vessels [30–32]. Nitroglycerin has a half-life of two minutes and is hydrolyzed by hepatic glutathione-organic nitrate reductase into inorganic nitrite and denitrated metabolites, which have little if any vasoactivity. In contrast to nitroprusside, tolerance develops rapidly to nitroglycerin and may result from impaired biotransformation.

Calcium Channel Blocker

Calcium channel blockers (CCBs) bind to L-type calcium channels located on vascular smooth muscle cells, cardiomyocytes, and cardiac nodal tissues, decreasing the influx of calcium into these cells. As a result, these agents thus induce vasodilation and may affect contractility, heart rate, and nodal conduction.

The most vascular-specific CCBs are the dihydropyridines, which include amlodipine, nifedipine, nicardipine, and isradipine. CCBs induce vasodilation of arterial and pulmonary resistance vessels, with no effect on venous capacitance vessels [33–35]. CCBs have been shown to have little if any effect on contractility [36, 37]. To the extent that a CCB has a direct effect on contractility, it is offset by a baroreceptor-mediated reflex activation of the sympathetic nervous system in response to vasodilation and a reduction in arterial blood pressure [33–37]. The overall hemodynamic effect is dominated by the reduction in peripheral resistance and ventricular afterload [33–37]. Of the CCBs, nicardipine is commonly used to acutely reduce arterial resistance and blood pressure. A continuous intravenous infusion of nicardipine has a half-life of 30–60 minutes, rendering it less titratable than other vasodilators such as nitroprusside. Clevidipine is a relatively new short-acting intravenous third-generation dihydropyridine CCB that has a shorter half-life of 15 minutes [38].

Vasopressin

Vasopressin is a peptide hormone synthesized in the hypothalamus and then transported to and stored in the pituitary gland. It is essential for osmotic and cardiovascular homeostasis. In addition to its antidiuretic effect, physiological levels of vasopressin are required for normal vascular tone. Vasopressin interacts with vasopressin-specific receptors located on vascular smooth muscle and renal tubular cells. Vasopressin vasoconstricts venous capacitance and systemic arterial resistance vessels in a dose-dependent fashion [10–13, 39–42]. Studies on the effects of vasopressin on the pulmonary circulation are mixed and may depend in part on the conditions [38–46]. Vasopressin does not appear to have an appreciable effect on pulmonary arterial resistance [43–48]. There is some evidence that vasopressin may increase the responsiveness of the vasculature to catecholamines [49, 50].

Conclusion

In this review, we discussed the impact of vasoactive agents used in the acute management of cardiac and vascular dysfunction. With establishment of and consideration given to the patient's hemodynamic phenotype, the selection of vasoactive therapy can then be based on which agent best addresses the physiologic derangement and is best suited to accomplish the therapeutic objectives. In doing so, one tailors therapies accordingly and avoids a formulaic approach to the management of critical cardiovascular disease.

References

1. Schwinn DA. Adrenoceptors and models for G protein-coupled receptors: structure, function and regulation. Br J Anaesth. 1993;71:77–85.
2. Feldman AM. Modulation of adrenergic receptors and G-transduction proteins in failing human ventricular myocardium. Circulation. 1993;87(suppl IV):IV-27-IV-34.
3. Floras JS. Sympathetic nervous system activation in human heart failure. J Am Coll Cardiol. 2009;54:375–85.
4. Driscoll DJ, Gillette PC, Duff DF, et al. The hemodynamic effect of dopamine in children. J Thorac Cardiovasc Surg. 1979;78:765–8.
5. Leier CV, Heban PT, Huss P, et al. Comparative systemic and regional hemodynamic effects of dopamine and dobutamine in patients with cardiomyopathic heart failure. Circulation. 1978;58:466–75.
6. Loeb HS, Bredakis J, Gunner RM. Superiority of dobutamine over dopamine for augmentation of cardiac output I patients with low output cardiac failure. Circulation. 1977;55:375–8.
7. Holloway EL, Stinson EB, Derby GC. Action of drugs in patients early after cardiac surgery. Comparison of isoproterenol and dopamine. Am J Cardiol. 1975;35:656–9.

8. Li J, Zhang G, Holtby H, et al. Adverse effects of dopamine on systemic hemodynamic status and oxygen transport in neonates after the Norwood procedure. J Am Coll Cardiol. 2006;48:1859–64.
9. Beregovich J, Bianchi C, Rubler S, et al. Dose-related hemodynamic and renal effects of dopamine in congestive heart failure. Am Heart J. 1974;87:550–7.
10. Greenway CV, Lautt WW. Effects of infusions of catecholamines, angiotensin, vasopressin and histamine on hepatic blood volume in the anaesthetized cat. Br J Pharmacol. 1972;44:177–84.
11. Pang C. Autonomic control of the venous system in health and disease: effects of drugs. Pharmacol Ther. 2001;90:179–230.
12. Arimura H, Bosnjak ZJ, Hoka S, et al. Catecholamine-induced changes in vascular capacitance and sympathetic nerve activity in dogs. Can J Physiol Pharmacol. 1992;70:1021–31.
13. Barman SA. Effect of catecholamines on pulmonary circulation at elevated vascular tone. J Appl Physiol. 1985;78:1452–8.
14. Hyman AL, Nandiwada P, Knight DS. Pulmonary vasodilator responses to catecholamines and sympathetic nerve stimulation in the cat. Circ Res. 1981;48:407–15.
15. Ducas J, Duval D, Dasilva H, et al. Treatment of canine pulmonary hypertension: effects of norepinephrine and isoproterenol on pulmonary vascular pressure-flow characteristics. Circulation. 1987;75:235–42.
16. Kersting F, Follath F, Moulds R, et al. A comparison of cardiovascular effects of dobutamine and isoprenaline after open heart surgery. Br Heart J. 1976;38:622–6.
17. Barrington K, Chan W. The circulatory effects of epinephrine infusion in the anesthetized piglet. Pediatr Res. 1993;33:190–4.
18. Stratton JR, Pfeifer MA, Ritchie JL, et al. Hemodynamic effects of epinephrine: concentration-effect study in humans. J Appl Physiol. 1985;58:1199–206.
19. Mackenzie SJ, Kapadia F, Nimmo GR, et al. Adrenaline in treatment of septic shock: effects of hemodynamics and oxygen transport. Intensive Care Med. 1991;17:36–9.
20. Moran JL, O'Fathartaigh MS, Peisach AR, et al. Epinephrine as an inotropic agent in septic shock: a dose-profile analysis. Crit Care Med. 1993;21:70–7.
21. Day N, Phu NH, Bethell DP, et al. The effects of dopamine and adrenaline infusions on acid-base balance and systemic haemodynamics in severe infection. Lancet. 1996;348:219–23.
22. Yamamoto K, Kodama K, Masuyama T, et al. Adverse effects of epinephrine in patients with advanced left ventricular dysfunction: analysis of ventriculo-arterial coupling. Int J Cardiol. 1992;32:143–55.
23. Lipman J, Roux A, Kraus P. Vasoconstrictor effects of adrenaline in human septic shock. Anaesth Intensive Care. 1991;19:61–5.
24. Rich S, Gubin S, Hart K. The effects of phenylephrine on right ventricular performance in patients with pulmonary hypertension. Chest. 1990;98:1102–6.
25. Chang AC, Atz AM, Wernovsky G, et al. Milrinone: systemic and pulmonary hemodynamic effects in neonates after cardiac surgery. Crit Care Med. 1995;23:1907–14.
26. Benotti JR, Lesko LJ, McCue JE, et al. Pharmacokinetics and pharmacodynamics of milrinone in chronic congestive heart failure. Am J Cardiol. 1985;56:685–9.
27. Young RA, Ward A. Milrinone—a preliminary review of its pharmacological properties and therapeutic use. Drugs. 1988;36:158–92.
28. Woolfrey SG, Hegbrant J, Thysell H, et al. Dose regimen adjustment for milrinone in congestive heart failure patients with moderate and severe renal failure. J Pharm Pharmacol. 1995;47:651–5.
29. Palmer RF, Lasseter KC. Sodium nitroprusside. N Engl J Med. 1975;292:294–7.
30. Ilbawi M, Isriss FS, DeLeon SY, et al. Hemodynamic effects of intravenous nitroglycerin in pediatric patients after heart surgery. Circulation. 1985;72(suppl II):II-101–7.
31. Hill NS, Antman EM, Green LH, et al. Intravenous nitroglycerin. Chest. 1981;79:69–76.
32. Miller RR, Vismara LA, Williams DO, et al. Pharmacological mechanisms for left ventricular unloading in clinical congestive heart failure. Circ Res. 1976;39:127–33.

33. Curran MP, Robinson DM, Keating GM. Intravenous nicardipine. Its use in the short-term treatment of hypertension and various other indications. Drugs. 2006;66:1755–82.
34. Visser CA, Koolen JJ, van Wezel H, et al. Hemodynamics of nicardipine in coronary artery disease. Am J Cardiol. 1987;59:9J–12J.
35. Singh BN, Josephson MA. Clinical pharmacology, pharmacokinetics, and hemodynamic effects of nicardipine. Am Heart J. 1990;119:427–34.
36. Tanaka K, Oshita S, Kitahata H, et al. Effects of nicardipine on ventriculo-arterial coupling in humans. Br J Anaesth. 1998;81:180–5.
37. Cheng C-P, Igarashi Y, Pettersson K, et al. Effect of felodipine on left ventricular performance in conscious dogs: assessment by left ventricular pressure-volume analysis. J Pharmacol Exp Ther. 1991;257:163–9.
38. Meeks ED, Keating GM, Keam SJ. Clevidipine: a review of its use in the management of acute hypertension. Am J Cardiovasc Drugs. 2009;9:117–34.
39. Holmes CL, Bm P, Russell JA, et al. Physiology of vasopressin relevant to the management of septic shock. Chest. 2001;120:989–100.
40. Jerath N, Frndova H, Gurofsky R, et al. Clinical impact of vasopressin infusion on hemodynamics, liver and renal function in pediatric patients. Intensive Care Med. 2008;34:1274–80.
41. Treschan TA, Peters J. The vasopressin system. Anesthesiology. 2006;105:599–612.
42. Goldsmith SR, Francis GS, Cowley AW Jr, et al. Hemodynamic effects of infused arginine vasopressin in congestive heart failure. J Am Coll Cardiol. 1986;8:779–83.
43. Evora PRB, Pearson PJ, Schaff HV. Arginine vasopressin induces endothelium-dependent vasodilation of the pulmonary artery. Chest. 1993;103:1241–5.
44. Tayama E, Ueda T, Shojima T, et al. Arginine vasopressin is an ideal drug after cardiac surgery for the management of low systemic vascular resistant hypotension concomitant with pulmonary hypertension. Interact Cardiovasc Thorac Surg. 2007;6:715–9.
45. Wallace AW, Tunin CM, Shoukas AA. Effects of vasopressin on pulmonary and systemic vascular mechanics. Am J Phys. 1989;257:H1228–34.
46. Eichinger MR, Walker BR. Enhanced pulmonary arterial dilation to arginine vasopressin in chronically hypoxic rats. Am J Phys. 1994;267:H2413–9.
47. Tsuneyoshi I, Yamada H, Kakihana Y, et al. Hemodynamic and metabolic effects of low-dose vasopressin infusions in vasodilatory septic shock. Crit Care Med. 2001;29:487–93.
48. Walker BR, Haynes J Jr, Wang HL, et al. Vasopressin-induced pulmonary vasodilation in rats. Am J Phys. 1989;257(2 Pt 2):H415–22.
49. Medina P, Noguera I, Aldasoro M, et al. Enhancement by vasopressin of adrenergic responses in human mesenteric arteries. Am J Phys. 1997;272:H1087–93.
50. Medina P, Acuna A, Martinez-Leon JN, et al. Arginine vasopressin enhances sympathetic constriction through the V1vasopressin receptor in human saphenous vein. Circulation. 1998;97:865–70.

Chapter 7
Hemodynamic Monitoring

Sebastian C. Tume, John M. Costello, and Ronald A. Bronicki

Introduction

Advanced hemodynamic monitoring is essential in the management of critically ill patients. It determines the hemodynamic phenotype, enabling the clinician to tailor therapies accordingly and to avoid a one-size-fits-all approach, to assess the response to interventions, and to establish a timely and accurate clinical trajectory. The assessment of cardiovascular function begins with physical examination and the interpretation of "standard" hemodynamic parameters such as heart rate, blood pressure, central venous pressure (CVP), and urine output. However, studies have demonstrated that estimations of cardiovascular function limited to this approach may be discordant from quantitative measurements [1–8]. These discrepancies have been shown to occur irrespective of clinical experience and medical training and in care of critically ill children and adults. The physical examination and the use of standard hemodynamic parameters are essential components of the clinical assessment of the critically ill patient. Advanced hemodynamic monitoring however may be necessary to establish an accurate and comprehensive physiologic profile, allowing for the implementation of a definitive management and resuscitative strategy.

S. C. Tume · R. A. Bronicki (✉)
Baylor College of Medicine, Texas Children's Hospital, Houston, TX, USA
e-mail: sctume@texaschildrens.org; rxbronic@texaschildrens.org

J. M. Costello
Medical University of South Carolina, Shawn Jenkins Children's Hospital, Charleston, SC, USA
e-mail: costello@musc.edu

R. A. Bronicki et al. (eds.), *Simulation in Cardiovascular Critical Care Medicine*, https://doi.org/10.1007/978-3-031-63557-1_7

Heart Rate

While heart rate does not provide an indication of cardiac output (CO) or the adequacy of tissue oxygenation, it is an important determinant of ventricular loading conditions, myocardial oxygen demand, and CO and thus contributes importantly to the underlying pathophysiology and impact of therapies.

Arterial Pressure

Being the product of CO and systemic vascular resistance (SVR), blood pressure varies in relation to changes in these two parameters and is thus not an indicator of CO. As with other hemodynamic parameters, blood pressure should be placed in its clinical context and used in conjunction with other monitoring modalities to create a comprehensive hemodynamic profile. Consensus generated goal systemic arterial blood pressure and coronary perfusion pressure for critically ill adult patients have been published [9]. Goal pressures for critically ill infants and children are less well defined [10].

An analysis of the arterial pulse pressure contributes to establishing a hemodynamic profile. The two primary factors that affect the pulse pressure are stroke volume and compliance or distensibility of the arterial circulation [11–18]. As resistance to peripheral blood flow increases, stroke volume decreases, and the pulse pressure narrows. Systolic and diastolic pressures rise, with the diastolic pressure rising to a greater extent. The opposite occurs with a decrease in arterial resistance. With a decrease in stroke volume resulting from a decrease in preload or contractility, the pulse pressure narrows; however, the systolic and diastolic pressures decrease. As arterial compliance decreases, the pulse pressure increases, with a rise in systolic pressure and a decrease in diastolic pressure. Heart rate also influences the pulse pressure. An isolated decrease in heart rate increases stroke volume and pulse pressure. In addition, as heart rate decreases, there is more time for pressure decay during diastole, which causes the diastolic pressure to decrease more than the systolic pressure. The opposite occurs with an increase in heart rate. Lesions that allow for aortic run-off during diastole increase the pulse pressure, including aortic insufficiency and an aorta to pulmonary artery communication.

Examination of the variation in arterial pressure that occurs during positive pressure ventilation provides insight into right ventricular (RV) loading conditions and function [19–24]. The physiologic underpinnings of this interaction are discussed in detail in Chap. 5. In brief, from an apneic baseline, as intrathoracic pressure (ITP) increases, the systolic transmural pressure for the thoracic arterial vessels decreases, and systemic arterial pressure rises (Fig. 7.1). After a cardiac cycle or two, the systolic pressure decreases, falling below the apneic baseline. This results from the effects of an increase in ITP on systemic venous return and RV preload and/or the impact of lung volume on RV afterload. In either case, the decrease in RV output

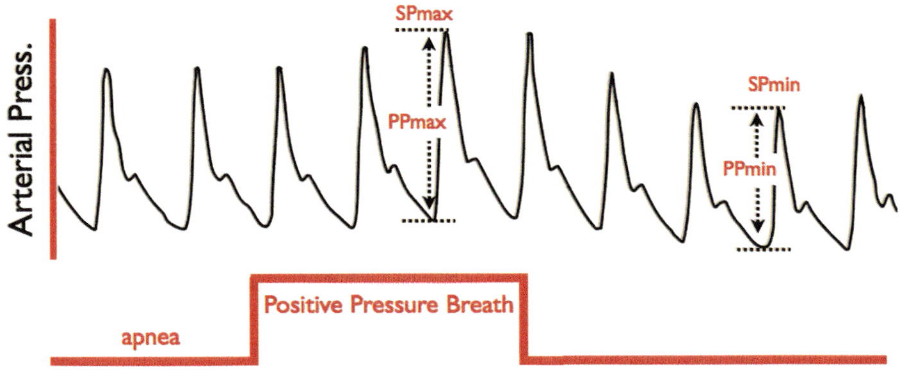

Fig. 7.1 *Variation in systemic arterial pressure during a positive pressure breath.* From an apneic baseline, as intrathoracic pressure rises, the systolic transmural pressure for the thoracic arterial vessels decreases, and as a result, the systemic arterial pressure increases. After a cardiac cycle or two, the systolic pressure decreases, falling below the apneic baseline. The rise in systolic pressure is referred to as the "maximum systolic pressure." The fall in systolic pressure is referred to as the "minimum systolic pressure." Systolic pressure variation (SPV) refers to the pressure gradient between the maximum and minimum systolic pressures. SPmax and SPmin denote maximal and minimal systolic arterial pressure, while PPmax and PPmin represent maximal and minimal pulse pressures

compromises left ventricular (LV) filling, stroke volume, and arterial pressure. The rise in systolic pressure is referred to as the "maximum systolic pressure." The fall in systolic pressure is referred to as the "minimum systolic pressure." Systolic pressure variation (SPV) refers to the pressure gradient between the maximum and minimum systolic pressures. Pulse pressure variation (PPV) is defined as the maximal pulse pressure less the minimum pulse pressure divided by the average of these two pressures. Quantifying the variation in pulse pressure with either the SPV or PPV indicates the degree to which RV stroke volume has been affected by alterations in ventricular loading conditions. Echocardiography provides invaluable information as to the mechanism(s) responsible [23–24].

Pulse Wave Analysis

CO can be estimated by analysis of the pulse contour from an arterial waveform. There are several systems available. Each relies on a unique computational algorithm [25–28] and assumptions and require calibration and periodic recalibration. These systems are less accurate in pediatric patients [27, 28].

Right Atrial Pressure

The right atrial pressure, a mean pressure measured throughout the cardiac cycle, is used as a surrogate for the RV end diastolic pressure (EDP) and in turn RV preload (end diastolic volume, EDV). Right and left atrial pressure waveforms (Fig. 7.2) normally demonstrate three positive and two negative waves: the "a" wave follows the p wave on the ECG and is produced by atrial contraction; the "c" wave is produced by ventricular contraction and bulging of the atrioventricular valve upward into the atrium; the "x" descent results from atrial relaxation and annual descent as the atrioventricular valve is pulled into the ventricle; the "v" wave results from atrial filling and occurs in late systole prior to opening of the atrioventricular valve; and the "y" descent results from opening of the atrioventricular valve and emptying of the atria.

A CVP equates with a right atrial pressure so long as the vena cava is under zone 3 conditions (see Chap. 5). A normal central venous or right atrial pressure is 2–5 mm Hg. Under normal conditions, the CVP approximates the RVEDP. However, in the presence of disease, it may not. With tricuspid stenosis, the CVP is elevated relative to the EDP. Tricuspid regurgitation raises the CVP above right atrial diastolic pressure and EDP and generates a "v" wave that equals RV systolic pressure. Cannon "a" waves are produced when right atrial contraction occurs against a stenotic or closed tricuspid valve as in tricuspid stenosis or atrioventricular disassociation. When RV stiffness is elevated, atrial systole generates an EDP that is disproportionately elevated relative to the CVP. In this case, the "a" wave provides an accurate measurement of the EDP. In addition, changes in RV stiffness alter the

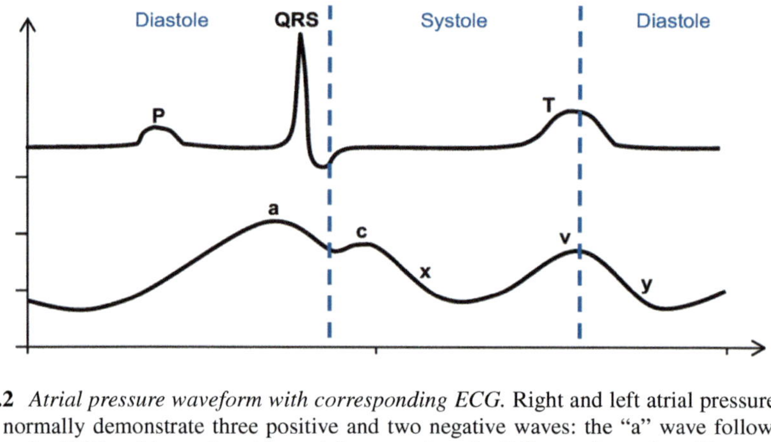

Fig. 7.2 *Atrial pressure waveform with corresponding ECG.* Right and left atrial pressure waveforms normally demonstrate three positive and two negative waves: the "a" wave follows the p wave on the ECG and is produced by atrial contraction; the "c" wave is produced by ventricular contraction and bulging of the atrioventricular valve upward into the atrium; the "x" descent results from atrial relaxation and annual descent as the atrioventricular valve is pulled into the ventricle; the "v" wave results from atrial filling and occurs in late systole prior to opening of the atrioventricular valve; and the "y" descent results from opening of the atrioventricular valve and emptying of the atria

relationship between the RV EDP and EDV, further confounding the relationship between the CVP and RV EDV [29]. Factors that decrease the effective compliance of the RV are pericardial disease and positive ITP. The latter is discussed in detail in Chap. 5.

Left Atrial Pressure and Pulmonary Artery Occlusion Pressure

The CVP does not provide an indication of, nor does it necessarily reflect, parallel changes in left atrial or LV EDP [30]. In 1970 Swan and Ganz first described the use of a balloon-tipped catheter inserted into the pulmonary artery for the measurement of the pulmonary artery occlusion pressure (PAOP) which in turn provides an indication of left atrial pressure [31–34]. This was soon followed by the implementation of a triple-lumen catheter with a thermistor tip that allowed for the measurement of CO by the thermodilution technique [31–34]. Heralded as a breakthrough in hemodynamic monitoring, the Swan-Ganz catheter or pulmonary arterial catheter (PAC) enabled the clinician to readily measure several hemodynamic variables that were not previously obtainable at the bedside. In addition to LV filling pressure, CO, and derivation of SVR, the PAC enables the clinician to measure pulmonary arterial pressure and mixed venous saturation and to derive pulmonary vascular resistance (PVR) and oxygen consumption.

Like the CVP, the PAOP is a mean pressure that is used as a surrogate for left atrial pressure and LV EDP and in turn LV EDV. However, these inferences are based on several assumptions which if incorrect lead to a misinterpretation of the data. The PAOP must be accurately measured, the PAOP must reflect left atrial pressure, the left atrial pressure must reflect the LV EDP, and this parameter must relate directly to the definition of preload, the EDV. Under normal conditions, the correlation between these parameters is very good. However, in the presence of cardiopulmonary disease, these parameters may be discordant from one another [35].

Vascular pressure equilibrates along a continuous column of blood that lacks flow, and thus the PAOP reflects left atrial pressure, and the balloon-tipped catheter generates similar atrial waveforms as the CVP tracing. For the PAOP to approximate left atrial pressure, a continuous column of blood must exist between the catheter tip and the left atrium (zone III conditions). With wedging, a tracing free of cardiac influences (loss of "a" and "v" waves) indicates non-zone III conditions, and the PAOP reflects changes in alveolar pressure rather than left atrial pressure.

The PAOP will be greater than the LV EDP in mitral stenosis and mitral regurgitation. In mitral regurgitation, the regurgitant volume increases the mean left atrial pressure above the diastolic left atrial pressure and EDP and generates an exaggerated "v" wave. A noncompliant left atrium will also generate a PAOP that is greater than the EDP. The PAOP will be greater than left atrial pressure and EDP in pulmonary vein stenosis. In pulmonary veno-occlusive disease (PVOD), there is no pressure gradient between the occluded pulmonary arterial catheter and left atrium, as flow resumes distal to the lesion (venules) [36]. The PAOP will be less than the EDP in aortic regurgitation and when LV stiffness is increased. In which case the "a" wave provides an accurate assessment of the EDP. And as is the case for the right heart, changes in ventricular or chamber stiffness alter the relationship between LV EDP and EDV, further confounding the relationship between the PAOP and LV EDV. Factors that decrease the effective compliance of the LV are pericardial disease and positive ITP.

Cardiac Output

A thermodilution-derived measurement of CO is based on the indicator dilution principle, which was first described by Stewart in the late 1800s and later refined by Hamilton. This involves injecting a volume of indicator into a central vein and observing the resultant change in concentration downstream over time. CO is determined by the amount of indicator divided by the change in concentration over time. Thermodilution involves injecting a known quantity volume of cold water into the right atrium and measuring the resultant temperature change with the thermistor located near the catheter tip. Using the Stewart-Hamilton equation, recording and displaying the temperature change from base line allows the calculation of blood flow with the area under the curve being inversely proportional to the CO. Studies have demonstrated thermodilution-derived CO measurements to be reliable in children and adults over a wide range of flows [37]. Pulmonary artery thermodilution-derived CO measurements remain accurate in the presence of left- or right-sided regurgitant lesions but are inaccurate in the setting of intracardiac shunt [38–42].

The transpulmonary thermodilution technique involves injection of the indicator in a central vein and relies on a thermistor in a proximal artery to measure the decrease in blood temperature. This method correlates very well with pulmonary artery thermodilution-derived measurements of CO and remains accurate in the presence of regurgitant right- or left-sided regurgitant lesions [43–49].

Echocardiography

Echocardiography is an essential diagnostic tool in the critical care setting, providing information on cardiovascular function and heart-lung interactions that is not available from other monitoring modalities. A detailed review of the use of echocardiography in the acute care setting is beyond the scope of this chapter [50]. Methodologies to assess ventricular systolic function such as the ejection fraction are sensitive to the arterial load. In the presence of tricuspid or mitral regurgitation, the respective ejection fraction overestimates contractility. Mitral and tricuspid inflow velocities and profiles provide an indication of diastolic function [51].

Diastolic ventricular dimensions give an indication of ventricular filling. Valvular function should be assessed. If valvular disease is present, imaging provides insight into the mechanisms responsible for dysfunction and importantly assesses the ventricular response and degree of compensation (chamber dimensions such as wall thickness and cavitary volume). Doppler technology may be used to measure intra- and extracardiac pressures, including pulmonary arterial systolic pressure, the presence and severity of a stenotic or regurgitant valve, and the presence and directionality of a septal defect and its potential impact on oxygenation. The ratio of RV to LV volume and the behavior and orientation of the interventricular septum during diastole and systole also contribute to establishing the pathophysiology and hemodynamic phenotype [51].

Venous Oximetry

The routine use of central venous catheters in the management of critically ill patients enables the clinician to apply the principles of venous oximetry and to assess oxygen extraction and the adequacy of tissue oxygenation. To accurately interpret and appreciate the use and limitations of venous oximetry requires an understanding of the determinants of tissue oxygenation; the relationship between oxygen consumption (VO_2) and oxygen delivery (DO_2); and global and regional compensatory circulatory responses to alterations in VO_2 and/or DO_2. This approach provides not only the physiologic underpinnings for interpretating venous oximetry and determining the adequacy of DO_2 but also a construct for defining the pathophysiology of shock states.

According to the Fick principle, total body VO_2 is equal to the product of CO and the difference in arterial—venous oxygen content ($CaO_2 - CvO_2$) or the volume of oxygen extracted per minute. Because oxygen is poorly soluble in water, the amount of oxygen dissolved in blood is minimal and inconsequential except in cases of severe anemia. By ignoring the amount of oxygen dissolved in blood, the Fick equation may be simplified and rearranged such that: $SaO_2 - SmvO_2 / SaO_2 = VO_2 / DO_2$, where DO_2 is the product of CO and arterial oxygen content; SaO_2 is the arterial oxygen saturation; $SmvO_2$ is the mixed venous oxygen saturation; and $SaO_2 - SmvO_2 / SaO_2$ is the oxygen extraction ratio (O_2ER). By assessing the O_2ER, the relationship between oxygen demand and DO_2 or oxygen transport balance can be assessed and the adequacy of tissue oxygenation determined.

If oxygen content is decreased, either due to impaired oxygenation or due to a decrease in the oxygen carrying capacity, CO increases, and a normal O_2ER is largely maintained [52–57]. With a more severe decrease in oxygen content and/or limitation in the compensatory increase in CO, oxygen extraction increases. Without a change in oxygen content or oxygen demand, as CO and thus DO_2 fall, oxygen extraction increases.

So long as the compensatory increase in oxygen extraction suffices, aerobic metabolism and VO_2 remain unchanged (the "oxygen supply independent" portion of the VO_2/DO_2 curve) (Fig. 7.3). Below a given DO_2, oxygen extraction continues to increase, but oxygen demand exceeds oxygen availability. At this point VO_2 falls, anaerobic metabolism ensures, and lactate begins to accumulate (the beginning of the "oxygen supply independent" portion of the VO_2/DO_2 curve) (Fig. 7.3). This represents the critical DO_2, which is the same regardless of whether the decrease in DO_2 resulted from anemia, hypoxemia, and or low CO [52–54]. The corresponding percent oxygen extraction represents the critical O_2ER. If oxygen requirements were to change, the critical DO_2 would change in parallel; however, the indicator of the adequacy of tissue oxygenation, the critical O_2ER remains constant between 60 and 70% [52–54]. The critical O_2ER also is unaffected by changes in the affinity of hemoglobin for oxygen (i.e., altered P50). Whether the P50 is decreased or increased [58, 59], the efficiency of oxygen extraction and the critical O_2ER remain unchanged.

Central Venous Oximetry

Alternative "central venous" sites for monitoring venous oximetry ($ScvO_2$) include the right atrium, the superior vena cava, the jugular vein, and the inferior vena cava-right atrial junction. The normal O_2ER for the superior vena cava is 25–30%, 30–35% for the jugular vein, and 15–20% for the right atria-inferior vena cava [60–65]. As CO and DO_2 fall, inferior vena cava saturations fall first, which is accompanied by a less severe drop in superior vena cava and right atrial SvO_2 as blood flow is redistributed away from less vital organs such as the kidneys and

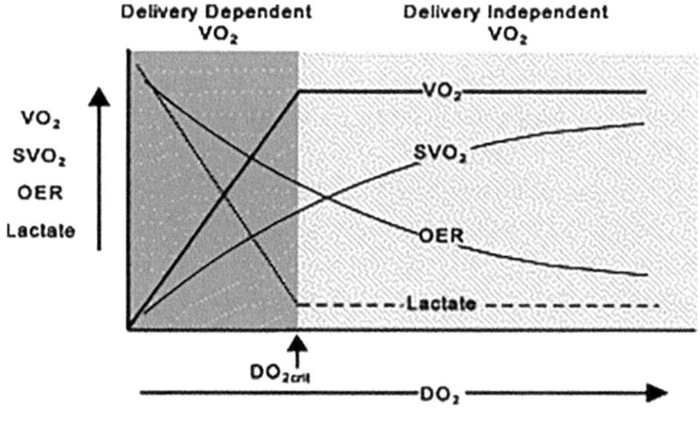

Fig. 7.3 *The relationship between oxygen delivery (DO_2) and oxygen consumption (VO_2).* For a given metabolic state, as DO_2 decreases, O_2 extraction and the oxygen extraction ratio (OER) increases, and VO_2 is maintained. As DO_2 decreases further, oxygen extraction continues to increase. At a given DO_2, the compensatory increase in oxygen extraction no longer suffices and VO_2 begins to decrease, which defines the onset of anaerobic metabolism and tissue hypoxia. The corresponding DO_2 represent the critical DO_2, while the corresponding OER represent the critical OER. As the OER rises above critical, lactate levels rise above the normal range, as the production of lactate outpaces its clearance. SvO_2, mixed venous oxygen saturation

mesentery. As CO and DO_2 fall further, the superior vena cava and right atrial SvO_2 begin to decrease [60–65].

In the presence of left-to-right intracardiac shunting, mixed venous oximetry is rendered useless, as is right atrial oximetry in the presence of left-to-right atrial shunting. Venous oximetry from the inferior vena cava may be useful if obtained from the right atrial junction; however, streaming does occur in the inferior vena cava. For superior vena cava and jugular venous oximetry, changes in the arterial PCO_2 will in the absence of changes in systemic perfusion alter the cerebral O_2ER, as cerebral blood flow is uncoupled from cerebral metabolism.

Advantages and Limitations of Venous Oximetry

It is not until the critical O_2ER is reached and the production of lactate exceeds its clearance that the serum lactate level begins to rise. Therefore, venous oximetry provides an indication of impending shock, while lactic acidosis is consistent with but not specific for a shock state.

A determination of CO and DO_2 does not provide an indication of whether they are adequate to meet metabolic demand. Oxygen demand may vary considerably between patients and change acutely for a given patient. There are several factors which impact oxygen demand, including body temperature, wakefulness, enteral nutrition, and respiratory load.

The O_2ER and changes in oxygen extraction do not necessarily reflect underlying cardiac function, CO, and DO_2, as changes in oxygen content and oxygen demand may vary.

The relationship between CO and venous oxygen saturations is curvilinear. Thus, for a given VO_2, venous oximetry is relatively insensitive at detecting changes in CO and DO_2 as they fall from normal values. It is when CO and DO_2 become low that further decreases produce a large increase in the O_2ER.

As alluded to above under central venous oximetry, global/systemic indicators of tissue oxygenation (VO_2/DO_2 relationship) do not necessarily reflect regional tissue oxygenation [66, 67]. For example, the critical O_2ER for the splanchnic circulation is similar to the global or systemic critical O_2ER. However, as CO falls, the splanchnic O_2ER increases first and becomes critical sooner than does the global O_2ER.

Conclusion

Standard hemodynamic monitoring does not reliably predict quantitative measures of cardiovascular function. Advanced hemodynamic monitoring establishes the hemodynamic phenotype, enabling the clinician to tailor therapies accordingly and to avoid a formulaic approach to care. This strategy establishes a timely and accurate clinical trajectory and allows for the development of a definitive management and resuscitative strategy.

References

1. Connors AF Jr, McCaffree DR, Gray BA. Evaluation of right-heart catheterization in the critically ill patient without acute myocardial infarction. N Engl J Med. 1983;308:263–7.
2. Tibby SM, Hatherill M, Murdoch IA. Capillary refill and core-peripheral temperature gap as indicators of haemodynamic status in paediatric intensive care patients. Arch Dis Child. 1999;80:163–6.
3. Tibby SM, Hatherill M, Marsh MJ, et al. Clinicians' abilities to estimate cardiac index in ventilated children and infants. Arch Dis Child. 1997;77:516–8.
4. Lobos AT, Lee S, Menon K. Capillary refill time and cardiac output in children undergoing cardiac catheterization. Pediatr Crit Care Med. 2012;13:136–40.
5. Steingrub JS, Celoria G, Vickers-Lahti M, et al. Therapeutic impact of pulmonary artery catheterization in a medical/surgical ICU. Chest. 1991;99:1451–5.
6. Eagle KA, Quertermous T, Singer DE, et al. Left ventricular ejection fraction. Physician estimates compared with gated blood pool scan measurements. Arch Intern Med. 1988;148:882–5.
7. Mattleman SJ, Hakki AH, Iskandrian AS, et al. Reliability of bedside evaluation in determining left ventricular function: correlation with left ventricular ejection fraction determined by radionuclide ventriculography. J Am Coll Cardiol. 1983;1:417–20.
8. Stevenson LW, Perloff JK. The limited reliability of physical signs for estimating hemodynamics in chronic heart failure. JAMA. 1989;261:884–8.
9. Cecconi M, De Backer D, Antonelli M, et al. Consensus on circulatory shock and hemodynamic monitoring. Task force of the European Society of Intensive Care Medicine. Intensive Care Med. 2014;40:1795–815.
10. Weiss SL, Peters MJ, Alhazzani W, et al. Surviving sepsis campaign international guidelines for the management of septic shock and sepsis-associated organ dysfunction in children. Pediatr Crit Care Med. 2020;21:e52–e106.
11. Stergiopulos N, Meister J-J, Westerhof N. Determinants of stroke volume and systolic and diastolic aortic pressure. Am J Phys. 1996;270:H2020–59.
12. Lamia B, Chemla D, Richard C, et al. Clinical review: interpretation of arterial pressure wave in shock states. Crit Care. 2005;9:601–6.
13. Augusto J-F, Teboul J-L, Radermacher P, et al. Interpretation of blood pressure signal: physiological basis, clinical relevance, and objectives during shock states. Intensive Care Med. 2011;37:411–9.
14. London GM, Pannier B. Arterial functions: how to interpret the complex physiology. Nephrol Dial Transplant. 2010;25:3815–23.
15. Westerhof N, Lankhaar J-W, Westerhof BE. The arterial Windkessel. Med Biol Eng Comput. 2009;47:131–41.
16. London GM, Guerin AP. Influence of arterial pulse and reflected waves on blood pressure and cardiac function. Am Heart J. 1999;138:S220–4.
17. Stergiopulos N, Westerhof N. Determinants of pulse pressure. Hypertension. 1998;32:556–9.
18. Madger SA. The highs and lows of blood pressure: toward meaningful clinical targets in patients with shock. Crit Care Med. 2014;42:1241–51.
19. Gunn SR, Pinsky MR. Implications of arterial pressure variation in patients in the intensive care unit. Curr Opin Crit Care. 2001;7:212–7.
20. Feihl F, Broccard AF. Interactions between respiration and systemic hemodynamics. Part II: practical implications in critical care. Intensive Care Med. 2009;35:198–205.

21. Monnet X, Teboul J-L. Assessment of fluid responsiveness: recent advances. Curr Opin Crit Care. 2018;24:190–5.
22. Magder S. Clinical usefulness of respiratory variations in arterial pressure. Am J Respir Crit Care Med. 2004;169:151–5.
23. Vieillard-Baron A, Loubieres Y, Schmitt JM, et al. Cyclic changes in right ventricular output impedance during mechanical ventilation. J Appl Physiol. 1999;87:1644–50.
24. Viellard-Baron A, Matthay M, Teboul JL. Experts' opinion on management of hemodynamics in ARDS patients: focus on the effects of mechanical ventilation. Intensive Care Med. 2016;42:739–49.
25. Saugel B, Kouz K, Scheeren T, et al. Cardiac output estimation using pulse wave analysis—physiology, algorithms, and technologies: a narrative review. Br J Anaesth. 2021;126:67–76.
26. Grensemann J. Cardiac output monitoring by pulse contour analysis, the technical basics of less-invasive techniques. Front Med. 2018;5:64.
27. Fakler U, Pauli C, Balling G, et al. Cardiac index monitoring by pulse contour analysis and thermodilution after pediatric cardiac surgery. J Thorac Cardiovasc Surg. 2007;133:224–8.
28. Mahajan A, Shabanie A, Turner J, et al. Pulse contour analysis for cardiac output monitoring in cardiac surgery for congenital heart disease. Anesth Analg. 2003;97:1283–8.
29. Reuse C, Vincent JL, Pinsky MR. Measurements of right ventricular volumes during fluid challenge. Chest. 1990;98:1450–4.
30. Forrester JS, Diamond G, McHugh TJ, et al. Filling pressures in the right and left sides of the heart in acute myocardial infarction. A reappraisal of central-venous-pressure monitoring. N Engl J Med. 1971;285:190–3.
31. Swan HJ, Ganz W, Forrester J, et al. Catheterization of the heart in man with use of a flow-directed balloon-tipped catheter. N Engl J Med. 1970;283:447–51.
32. Ganz W, Donoso R, Marcus HS, et al. A new technique for measurement of cardiac output by thermodilution in man. Am J Cardiol. 1971;27:392–6.
33. Forrester JS, Ganz W, McHugh T, et al. Thermodilution cardiac output determination with a single flow-directed catheter. Am Heart J 1972; 83:306–11.
34. Forrester JS. A tale of serendipity, ingenuity, and chance. J Am Coll Cardiol. 2019;74:100–3.
35. Raper R, Sibbald WJ. Misled by the wedge? The Swan-Ganz catheter and left ventricular preload. Chest. 1986;89:427–34.
36. Mandel J, Mark EJ, Hales CA. Pulmonary veno-occlusive disease. Am J Respir Crit Care Med. 2000;162:1964–73.
37. Moodie DS, Feldt RH, Kaye MP, et al. Measurement of postoperative cardiac output by thermodilution in pediatric and adult patients. J Thorac Cardiovasc Surg. 1979;78:796–8.
38. Hillis LD, Firth BG, Winniford MD. Comparison of thermodilution and indocyanine green dye in low cardiac output or left-sided regurgitation. Am J Cardiol. 1986;57:1201–2.
39. Hillis LD, Firth BG, Winniford MD. Analysis of factors affecting the variability of Fick versus indicator dilution measurements of cardiac output. Am J Cardiol. 1985;56:764–8.
40. Hoeper MM, Maier R, Tongers J, et al. Determination of cardiac output by the Fick method, thermodilution, and acetylene rebreathing in pulmonary hypertension. Am J Respir Crit Care Med. 1999;160:535–41.
41. Cigarroa RG, Lange RA, Williams RH, et al. Underestimation of cardiac output by thermodilution in patients with tricuspid regurgitation. Am J Med. 1989;86:417–20.
42. Boerboom LE, Kinney TE, Olinger GN, et al. Validity of cardiac output measurement by the thermodilution method in the presence of acute tricuspid regurgitation. J Thorac Cardiovasc Surg. 1993;106:636–42.
43. Proulx F, Lemson J, Choker G, et al. Hemodynamic monitoring by transpulmonary thermodilution and pulse contour analysis in critically ill children. Pediatr Crit Care Med. 2011;12:459–66.
44. Tibby SM, Hatherill M, Marsh MJ, et al. Clinical validation of cardiac output measurements using femoral artery thermodilution with direct Fick in ventilated children and infants. Intensive Care Med. 1997;23:987–91.

45. Pauli C, Fakler U, Genz T, et al. Cardiac output determination in children: equivalence of the transpulmonary thermodilution method to the direct Fick principle. Intensive Care Med. 2002;28:947–52.
46. Monnet X, Tebout J-L. Transpulmonary thermodilution: advantages and limits. Crit Care. 2017;21:147.
47. Breukers R-M, Groeneveld AB, de Wilde R, et al. Transpulmonary versus continuous thermodilution cardiac output after valvular and coronary artery surgery. Interact Cardiovasc Thorac Surg. 2009;9:4–8.
48. Staier K, Wilhelm M, Wiesenack C, et al. Pulmonary artery vs. transpulmonary thermodilution for the assessment of cardiac output in mitral regurgitation: a prospective observational study. Eur J Anaesthesiol. 2012;29:431–7.
49. Petzoldt M, Trepte CJ, Ridder J, et al. Reliability of transcardiopulmonary thermodilution cardiac output measurement in experimental aortic valve insufficiency. PLoS One. 2017;12(10):e0186481.
50. Rudski LG, Gargani L, Armstrong WF, et al. Stressing the cardiopulmonary vascular system: the role of echocardiography. J Am Soc Echocardiogr. 2018;31:527–50.
51. Cortes-Puentes GA, Oeckler RA, Marini JJ. Physiology-guided management of hemodynamics in acute respiratory distress syndrome. Ann Transl Med. 2018;6(18):353.
52. Cain SM. Oxygen delivery and uptake in dogs during anemic and hypoxic hypoxia. J Appl Physiol. 1977;42:228–34.
53. Dantzker DR, Foresman B, Gutierrez G. Oxygen supply and utilization relationships. A reevaluation. Am Rev Respir Dis. 1991;143:675–9.
54. Baigorri F, Russell JA. Oxygen delivery in critical illness. Crit Care Clin. 1996;12:971–94.
55. Woodson RD, Wills RE, Lenfant C. Effect of acute and established anemia on O_2 transport at rest, submaximal and maximal work. J Appl Physiol. 1978;44:36–43.
56. Vincent JL. Determination of oxygen delivery and consumption versus cardiac index and oxygen extraction ratio. Crit Care Clin. 1996;12:995–1006.
57. Cain SM. Peripheral oxygen uptake and delivery in health and disease. Clin Chest Med. 1983;4:139–48.
58. Schumacker PT, Long GR, Wood LD. Tissue oxygen extraction during hypovolemia: role of hemoglobin p50. J Appl Physiol. 1987;62:1801–7.
59. Curtis SE, Walker TA, Bradley WE, et al. Raising p50 increases tissue PO_2 in canine skeletal muscle but does not affect critical O_2 extraction ratio. J Appl Physiol. 1997;83:1681–9.
60. Lee J, Wright F, Barber R, et al. Central venous oxygen saturation in shock: a study in man. Anesthesiology. 1972;36:472–8.
61. Davies GG, Mendenhall J, Symreng T. Measurement of right atrial oxygen saturation by fiberoptic oximetry accurately reflects mixed venous oxygen saturation in swine. J Clin Monit. 1988;4:99–102.
62. Perez AC, Eulmesekian PG, Minces PG, et al. Adequate agreement between venous oxygen saturation in right atrium and pulmonary artery in critically ill children. Pediatr Crit Care Med. 2009;10:76–9.
63. Reinhart K, Rudolph T, Bredle DL, et al. Comparison of central-venous to mixed-venous oxygen saturation during changes in oxygen supply/demand. Chest 1989; 95:1216–21.
64. Barratt-Boyes BG, Wood EH. The oxygen saturation of blood in the venae cavae, right-heart chambers, and pulmonary vessels of healthy subjects. J Lab Clin Med. 1957;50:93–106.
65. Scheinman MM, Brown MA, Rapaport E. Critical assessment of use of central venous oxygen saturation as a mirror of mixed venous oxygen in severely ill cardiac patients. Circulation. 1969;40:165–72.
66. Nelson DP, King CE, Dodd SL, et al. Systemic and intestinal limits of O_2 extraction in the dog. J Appl Physiol. 1987;63:387–94.
67. Dahn MS, Lange MP, Jacobs LA. Central mixed and splanchnic venous oxygen saturation monitoring. Intensive Care Med. 1988;14:373–8.

Chapter 8
Acute Left Ventricular Systolic Heart Failure

Saul Flores, Rohit S. Loomba, and Ronald A. Bronicki

There are several processes that cause acute left ventricular (LV) systolic heart failure including arrhythmias, valvular disease, acute coronary syndrome, progression of chronic heart failure, and myocarditis. Regardless of the precipitating event, the common denominator is a limited stroke volume and cardiac output and pulmonary venous hypertension-induced lung injury and dysfunction.

Treatment begins with identifying and addressing reversible causes of heart failure. Neurohormonal activation contributes significantly to the pathophysiology and syndrome of acute LV systolic heart failure by altering LV loading conditions. Constriction of venous capacitance vessels and an increase in total blood volume increase the stressed blood volume (see Chap. 5). Constriction of systemic arterial resistance vessels increases LV afterload, which, coupled with a decrease in LV contractility, increases the end systolic volume. As a result of these changes, the LV end diastolic volume and pressure increase significantly, producing cardiogenic pulmonary edema (see Chap. 5) [1, 2]. Exaggerated negative pressure breathing contributes to an increase in LV loading conditions (see Chap. 5). The decrease in lung compliance and metabolic acidosis-induced increase minute ventilation increases respiratory muscle oxygen consumption (VO_2). The rise in LV diastolic pressure decreases the coronary perfusion pressure gradient (aortic diastolic pressure—LV diastolic pressure), while an increase in myocardial VO_2 shifts the lower inflection

S. Flores · R. A. Bronicki (✉)
Baylor College of Medicine, Texas Children's Hospital, Houston, TX, USA
e-mail: sxflore5@texaschildrens.org; rxbronic@texaschildrens.org

R. S. Loomba
Chicago Medical School/Rosalind Franklin University of Medicine, Advocate Children's Hospital, Chicago, IL, USA
e-mail: rohit.loomba@advocatehealth.com

R. A. Bronicki et al. (eds.), *Simulation in Cardiovascular Critical Care Medicine*, https://doi.org/10.1007/978-3-031-63557-1_8

point of the coronary pressure autoregulation curve up and to the right (as does a decrease in arterial oxygen content), indicating that myocardial ischemia develops at a higher coronary arterial pressure (Fig. 8.1) [3–5].

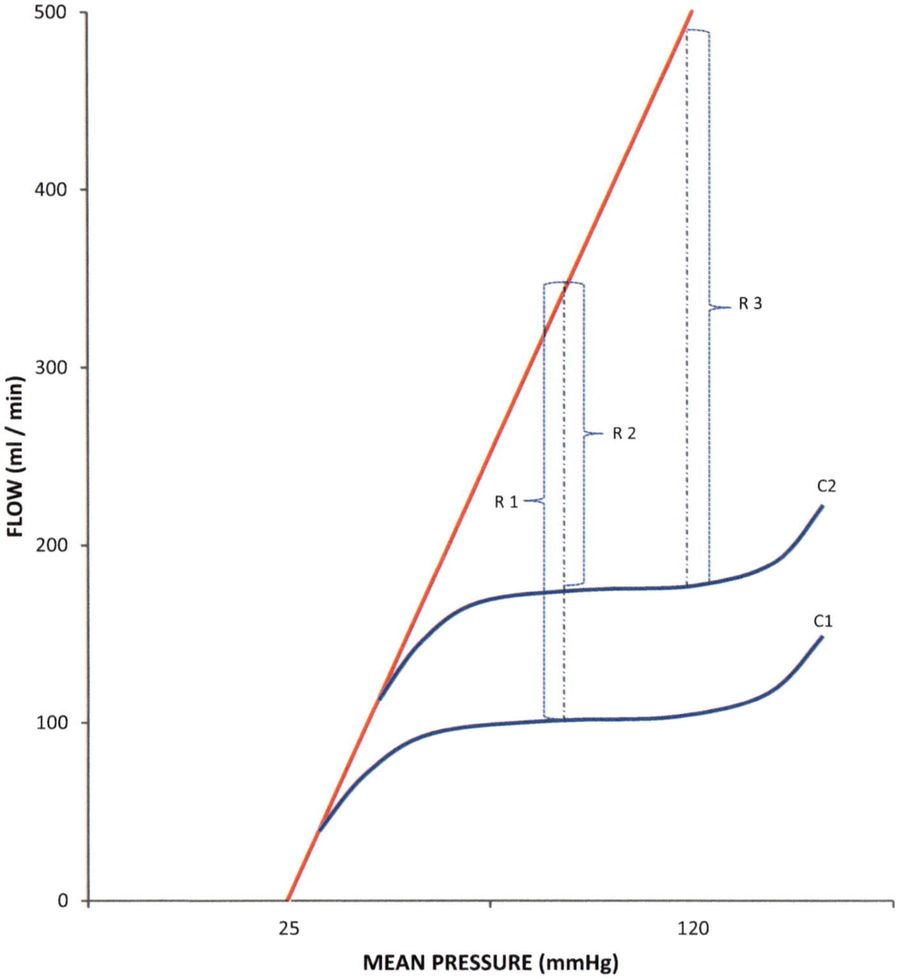

Fig. 8.1 *Coronary pressure autoregulation and coronary flow reserve*. Coronary flow is independent of coronary pressure over a wide range of pressures. Above or below the upper and lower inflection points, flow becomes pressure passive because at these pressures maximal vasoconstriction and vasodilation have occurred. C1 represents a normal LV, where C2 represents a LV that has elevated baseline flow and thus DO_2 due to either a decrease in arterial oxygen content (anemia or hypoxemia) or increase in oxygen demand. For a given coronary pressure, flow is greater for C2 than for C1. Thus, C2 has reduced coronary flow reserve (R2 < R1). With an increase in the perfusion pressure, coronary flow reserve increases (R3 > R2). Conversely, elevated LV diastolic pressure decreases coronary flow reserve

Positive airway pressure not only recruits and maintains end expiratory lung volume and improves oxygenation but has significant beneficial effects on LV loading conditions. As a result, cardiac output improves, and myocardial and respiratory pump VO_2 are reduced [6, 7].

Advanced hemodynamic monitoring should be considered to establish the hemodynamic phenotype, enabling the clinician to tailor therapies accordingly, and to assess the response to therapies. Vasoactive therapy may suffice in resuscitating and maintaining adequate cardiovascular function or serve as a bridge to mechanical circulatory support.

There is no consensus on the optimal vasoactive regimen to treat acute LV systolic heart failure in children or adults [8–12]. The 2022 statement of The American Heart Association (AHA) on pediatric myocarditis recommends an inodilator such as milrinone as the first-line agent unless the patient is hypotensive in which case an inoconstrictor is recommended [8]. The 2020 international consensus statement on cardiopulmonary resuscitation and emergency cardiovascular care in children published in Circulation makes the following recommendation: "It is reasonable to use epinephrine, levosimendan, dopamine or dobutamine for inotropic support in infants and children with cardiogenic shock [9]." The most recent statements from the AHA on adult myocarditis published in 2022 and adult cardiogenic shock published in 2017 emphasize the use of inoconstrictors such as norepinephrine and dopamine and in some cases a vasopressor such as arginine vasopressin or phenylephrine depending on the underlying cause and hemodynamic phenotype [10, 11].

With these broad recommendations in mind, we use the elastance model and ventricular pressure-volume relationship to illustrate the impact of an inoconstrictor/vasoconstrictor strategy and contrast it with an inodilator/vasodilator strategy in the care of a patient with acute LV systolic heart failure (Figs. 8.2, 8.3, 8.4, 8.5, and 8.6). The emphasis is on the *effects* of each agent on the circulation and in turn pressure and flow rather than the *agent or class of agent* selected. The changes in magnitude of the hemodynamic parameters may vary depending on the host response to the therapy.

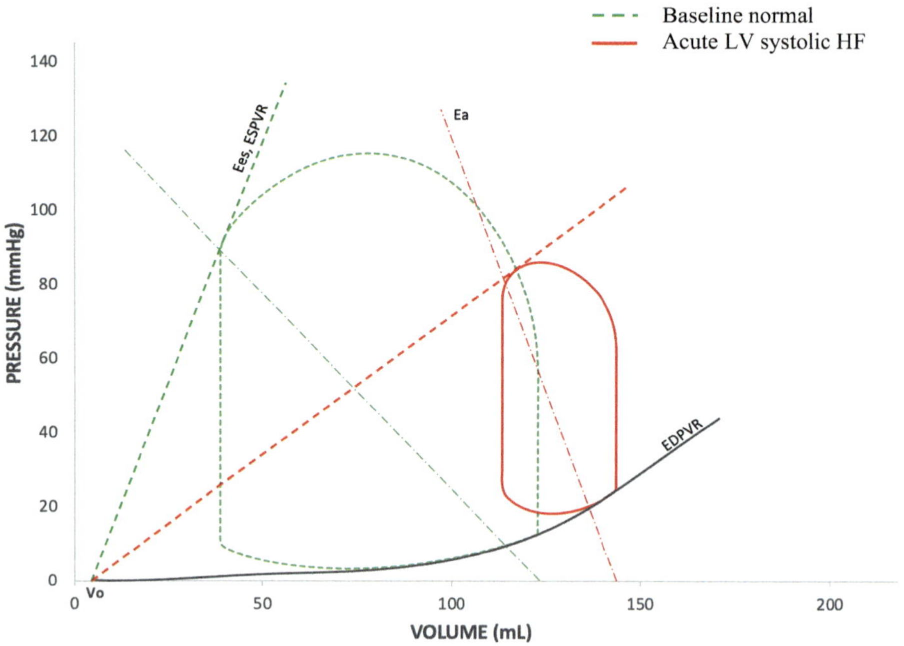

Fig. 8.2 *Acute LV systolic HF.* These PVLs illustrate the development of acute LV systolic HF in an adolescent patient. LV Ees is severely decreased, which has led to neurohormonal activation and increase in HR and SVR. As a result of the increase in HR and SVR, Ea is significantly elevated. The marked increase in Ea/Ees significantly reduces the EF and SV and increases the ESV. The decrease in Pes is limited as the decrease in Ees is partially offset by the increase in Ea. The significant decrease in SV has narrowed the pulse pressure, which is characterized by an increase in diastolic pressure, decrease in systolic pressure and maintained mean BP. The EDV and EDP are elevated due to the increase in ESV coupled with neurohormonal activation-induced venoconstriction and increase in SBV and in turn systemic venous return (see Chap. 5). The significantly elevated EDP leads to cardiogenic pulmonary edema

In acute LV systolic HF, the increase in EDV is relatively limited. This contrasts with chronic LV systolic HF where ventricular remodeling leads to significant chamber enlargement and large increase in EDV

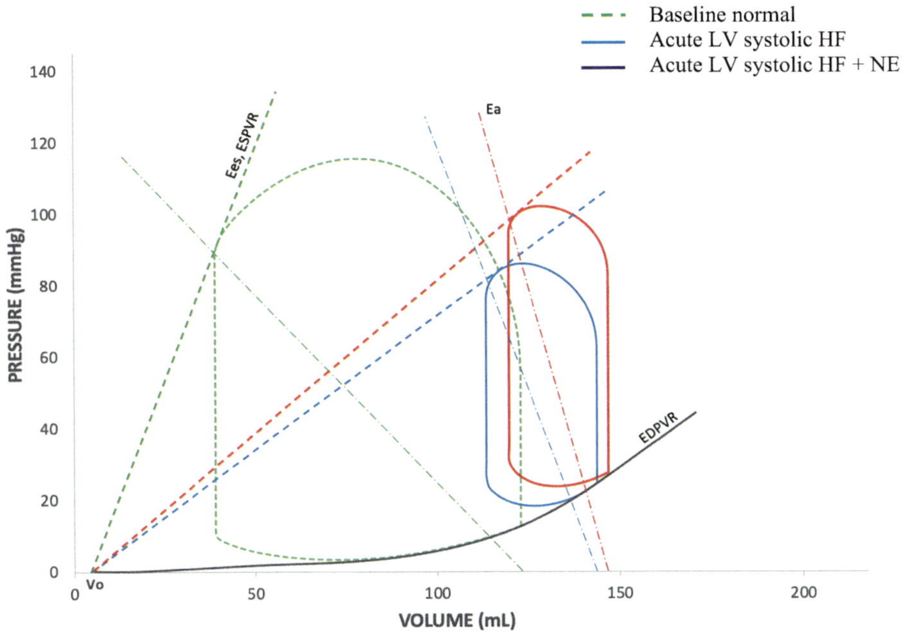

Fig. 8.3 *Impact of an inoconstrictor in acute LV systolic HF.* The inoconstrictor NE increases Ea and to a lesser extent Ees, the former due to a significant increase in SVR and to a lesser extent HR [13]. LV Ea/Ees has increased, worsening ventricular arterial uncoupling. As a result, the EF and SV have decreased further, the ESV has increased. Because Ea and Ees have both increased, Pes, as well as mean and systolic pressure, have increased considerably. The EDV and EDP have increased due to the increase in ESV coupled with NE-induced venoconstriction and increase in SBV. While the increase in EDV was limited, the EDP increased appreciably due to the marked increase in operating stiffness. Despite the increase in LV EDP, the CPP has become adequate due to the greater increase in aortic diastolic pressure

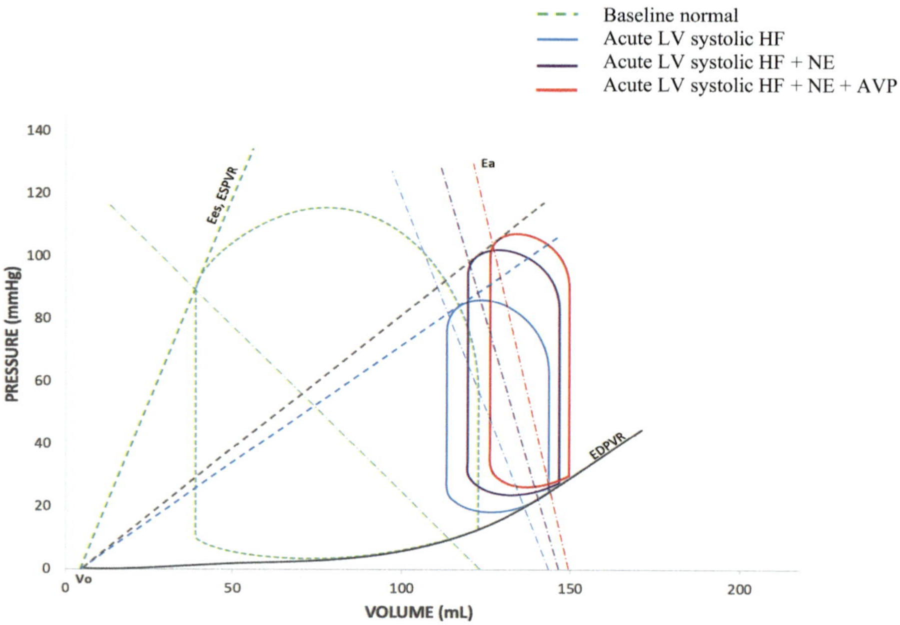

Fig. 8.4 *Impact of the inoconstrictor (NE) plus vasopressor in acute LV systolic HF.* The vasopressor AVP further vasoconstricts venous capacitance and arterial resistance vessels. The increase in SVR increases Ea and Ea/Ees and the extent of ventricular arterial uncoupling. The EF and SV decrease further, the ESV increases. The increase in Ea further increases the Pes. As with NE, the EDV and EDP increase due to the increase in ESV coupled with AVP-induced venoconstriction and increase in SBV. And while the increase in EDV was limited, the significant increase in operating stiffness leads to a further increase in EDP

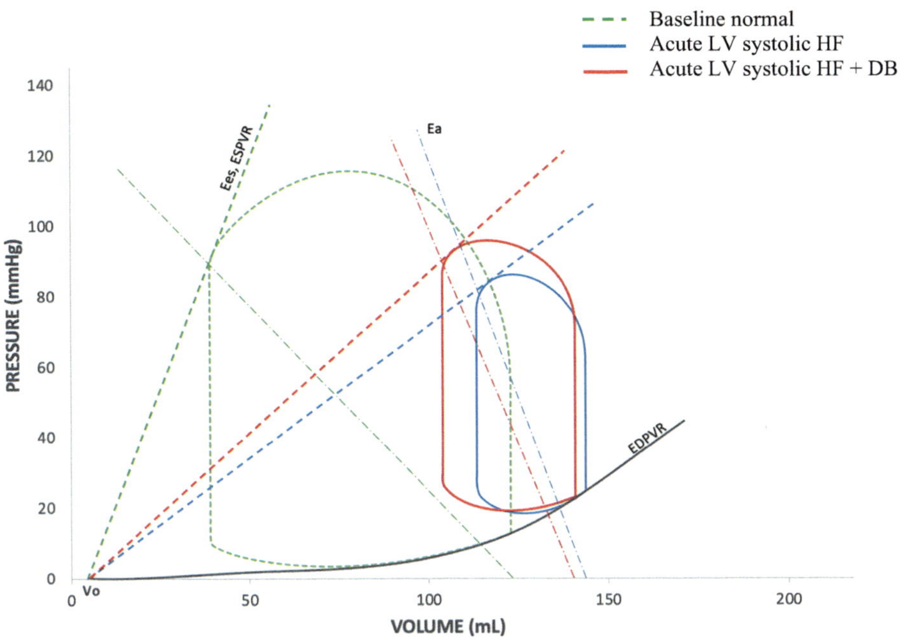

Fig. 8.5 *Impact of an inodilator in acute LV systolic HF.* The inodilator DB was titrated to increase LV Ees to a similar degree as occurred with NE. In this instance, Ea decreased because SVR decreased to a greater extent than HR increased. The net effect is a decrease in Ea/Ees, which improves ventricular arterial coupling, the EF and SV. Because Ees increases to a greater extent than Ea decreases, Pes, as well as mean and systolic BP, increase. The arterial load (Ea) has decreased; however, despite its vasodilatory properties, LV afterload has increased (systolic BP). In contrast to NE, DB decreases the ESV and SBV (venodilation), causing the EDV and EDP to decrease

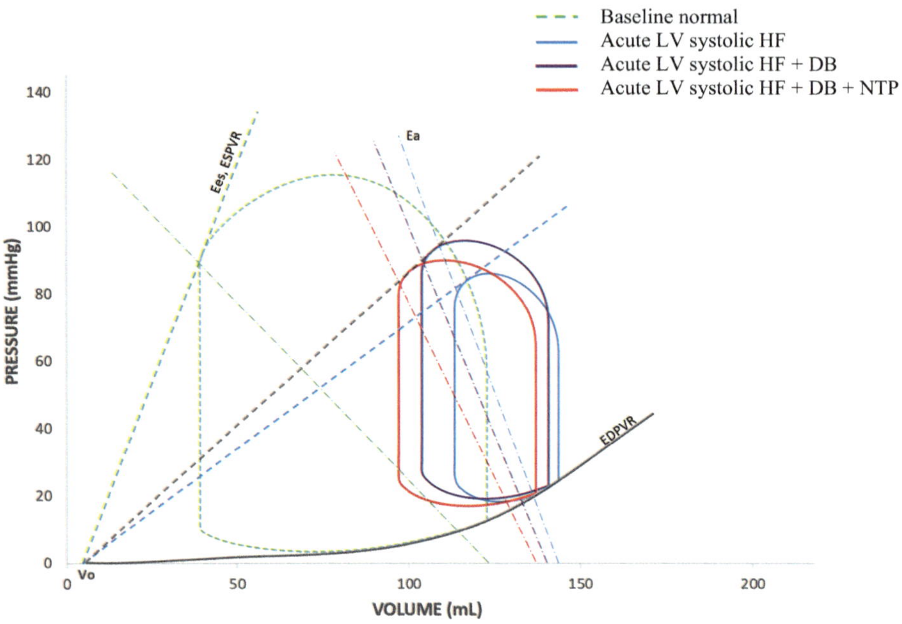

Fig. 8.6 *Impact of the inodilator (DB) plus a vasodilator.* The vasoactive agent NTP vasodilates venous capacitance and arterial resistance vessels. By decreasing SVR, Ea/Ees decreases, the EF and SV increase further. Ees is unaffected, Ea decreases and thus Pes decreases. The arterial load and LV afterload are both reduced. The decrease in ESV coupled with venodilation and reduction in SBV cause the EDV and EDP to decrease further
When comparing the inodilator plus vasodilator to inoconstrictor plus vasoconstrictor strategy, with similar increases in LV Ees and HR for each, the former resulted in a 1.5-fold greater CO and one-third lower EDP, with much greater mechanical efficiency (SW/PVA) and reduced myocardial VO_2 (see Chap. 2). While the perfusion pressures were lower, they were adequate with a mean aortic pressure and CPP of 76 and 45 mmHg, respectively

References

1. Burkhoff D, Tyberg JV. Why does pulmonary venous pressure rise after onset of LV dysfunction: a theoretical analysis. Am J Phys. 1993;265:H1819–28.
2. Magder S, Veerassamy S, Bates JHT. A further analysis of why pulmonary venous pressure rises after onset of LV dysfunction. J Appl Physiol. 2009;106:81–90.
3. Duncher DJ, Koller A, Cantry JM Jr. Regulation of coronary blood flow in health and ischemic heart disease. Prog Cardiovasc Dis. 2015;57:409–22.
4. Tune JD, Goodwill AG, Kiel AM, et al. Disentangling the Gordian know of local metabolic control of coronary blood flow. Am J Physiol Heart Circ Physiol. 2020;318:H11–24.
5. Van de Hoef TP, Nolte F, Rolandi MC, et al. Coronary pressure-flow relations as basis for the understanding of coronary physiology. J Mol Cell Cardiol. 2012;52:786–93.
6. Bradley TD, Holloway RM, McLaughlin PR, et al. Cardiac output response to continuous positive airway pressure in congestive heart failure. Am Rev Respir Dis. 1992;145:377–82.
7. Masip J, Roque M, Sanchez B, et al. Noninvasive ventilation in acute cardiogenic pulmonary edema. JAMA. 2005;294:3124–30.

8. Law YM, Lal AK, Chen S, et al. Diagnosis and management of myocarditis in children. A scientific statement from the American Heart Association. Circulation. 2021;1(144):e123–35.
9. Maconochie IK, Aickin R, Hazinski MF, et al. Pediatric life support. 2020 international consensus on cardiopulmonary resuscitation and emergency cardiovascular care science with treatment recommendations. Circulation. 2020;142(suppl 1):S140–84.
10. Kociol RD, Cooper LT, Fang JC, et al. Recognition and initial management of fulminant myocarditis. A scientific statement from the American Heart Association. Circulation. 2020;141:e69–92.
11. van Diepen S, Katz JN, Albert NM, et al. Contemporary management of cardiogenic shock. A scientific statement from the American Heart Association. Circulation. 2017;136:e232–68.
12. Levy B, Bastien O, Bendjelid K, et al. Experts' recommendations for the management of adult patients with cardiogenic shock. Ann Intensive Care. 2015;5(17):1–10.
13. Hollenberg SM. Vasoactive drugs in circulatory shock. Am J Respir Crit Care Med. 2011;183:847–55.

Chapter 9
Chronic Left Ventricular Systolic Heart Failure

Kriti Puri, Kyle D. Hope, and Daniel J. Penny

Chronic, dilated left ventricular (LV) systolic heart failure may result from many causes, including familial (genetic) cardiomyopathy, coronary insufficiency, myocarditis, valvular disease, and arrhythmia. Although the initiating cause may vary, they share similar molecular, biochemical, and mechanical processes that lead to LV eccentric remodeling and the chronic systolic heart failure phenotype.

As LV contractility wanes, LV end diastolic volume and pressure and mechanical stress increase. Neurohormonal activation contributes to the hemodynamic load by further increasing the volume and pressure load on the LV. An increase in systemic vascular resistance increases the arterial load, while venoconstriction and intravascular volume expansion combine to increase the stressed blood volume and systemic venous return [1]. The innate immune system is activated, which in conjunction with biomechanical and neurohormonal signaling, induces changes in gene expression and the structure and composition of cardiomyocyte and extracellular matrix. These processes result in changes in LV size, structure, and function [2–8]. The LV becomes markedly dilated and spherical in shape. Contractility deteriorates, myocardial relaxation is impaired, and diastolic stiffness is reduced.

Persistently elevated ventricular volume and pressure and neurohormonal activation drive the process of ventricular remodeling, leading to progressive increases in LV size and further reductions in systolic function. These findings contrast with those seen in patients with acute impairments in LV contractility, where ventricular remodeling has not occurred and ventricular dilation is limited.

K. Puri (✉) · K. D. Hope · D. J. Penny
Baylor College of Medicine, Texas Children's Hospital, Houston, TX, USA
e-mail: kxpuri@texaschildrens.org; kyle.hope@bcm.edu; djpenny@texaschildrens.org

R. A. Bronicki et al. (eds.), *Simulation in Cardiovascular Critical Care Medicine*, https://doi.org/10.1007/978-3-031-63557-1_9

In chronic LV systolic heart failure, marked ventricular dilation may impair leaflet coaptation of an otherwise structurally normal mitral valve, leading to secondary or functional mitral regurgitation [9–13]. This may be exacerbated as LV enlargement leads to displacement of papillary muscles resulting in tethering and restricted leaflet closure of the mitral valve leaflets. Ischemia or infarction of the papillary muscles may additionally contribute to impaired leaflet coaptation. Mitral regurgitation limits forward stroke volume and cardiac output and contributes to pulmonary venous hypertension. In contrast to primary mitral regurgitation, secondary mitral regurgitation is dynamic in nature. Changes in ventricular loading conditions, size, and shape may alter the regurgitant orifice area [11–13]. Given the vicious cycle of worsening cardiac function leading to increased mitral regurgitation and vice versa, it is often difficult in the clinical setting to determine the relative contributions of impaired contractility and functional mitral regurgitation to patient phenotype.

Acute LV systolic heart failure with or without secondary mitral regurgitation elevates pulmonary venous pressure, which increases the formation of extravascular lung water and may lead to alveolar edema and impaired oxygenation. Chronic pulmonary venous hypertension however induces compensatory changes within the pulmonary microvasculature and lung lymphatics, which limit the accumulation of extravascular lung water [14–18]. Pulmonary lymphatics become functionally hypertrophied, and changes occur to the alveolar-capillary barrier which increase the filtration threshold. For these reasons, despite a significantly elevated pulmonary microvascular hydrostatic pressure, the accumulation of extravascular lung water is limited, and oxygenation is not impaired [19]. Nonetheless, if hydrostatic pressure were to rise acutely from an elevated baseline, extravascular lung water would accumulate, leading to interstitial edema and, if severe enough, alveolar edema and impaired oxygenation [19].

Pulmonary venous hypertension also increases pulmonary arterial pressure and right ventricular (RV) afterload. Chronic pulmonary venous hypertension may induce pulmonary vascular remodeling and heightened pulmonary vascular reactivity, each of which contributes to further increases in pulmonary vascular resistance and pulmonary arterial pressure and RV afterload [20].

The pressure volume loops shown here (Figs. 9.1, 9.2, 9.3, 9.4, 9.5, 9.6, and 9.7) illustrate the progression from acute LV systolic failure and cardiogenic shock to chronic compensated (remodeled) systolic heart failure to acute deterioration of chronic systolic heart failure. This is followed by a set of pressure volume loops and hemodynamic data that illustrate the development of chronic compensated and decompensated LV systolic heart failure and functional mitral regurgitation (Figs. 9.8, 9.9, 9.10, and 9.11).

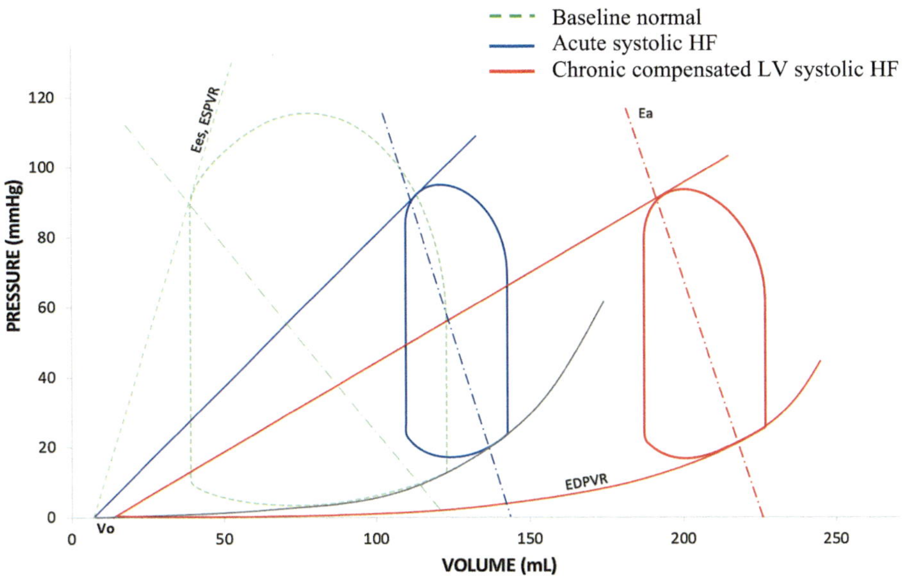

Fig. 9.1 *Chronic compensated LV systolic HF*. These PVLs illustrate the progression from normal LV function and loading conditions to the development of acute LV systolic HF and cardiogenic shock to the development of chronic compensated LV systolic HF in an adolescent patient. Following the insult to the myocardium and the development of acute LV systolic HF, contractility has decreased further and is reflected in a decrease in the ESPVR and a shift of Vo to the right (see Chap. 2). Ventricular remodeling has led to significant LV chamber enlargement and a decrease in LV chamber stiffness, which is reflected in a shift of the EDPVR down and to the right. Despite the marked increase in EDV, the EDPs for the acute and chronic states are similar. Chronic left atrial hypertension has led to compensatory adaptative changes within the lung such that extent of extravascular lung water formation is limited and normal oxygenation is preserved. Compared to the acute state, Ea has decreased somewhat due to a modest decrease in SVR and HR, however, ventricular-arterial uncoupling has increased as Ees has decreased to a greater extent than Ea. Despite this, the SV has increased due to the marked increase in EDV

The recommendations from consensus-driven statements on the care of children and adults with critical heart failure and cardiogenic shock vary considerably [21–23]. Recommendations for front-line vasoactive agents include inodilators, inoconstrictors, and vasopressors. For these reasons, we have contrasted the impact of these agents in patients with varying hemodynamic profiles. The emphasis is on the *effects* of each agent on the circulation and in turn pressure and flow rather than the *agent or class of agent* selected. The changes in magnitude of the hemodynamic parameters may vary depending on the host response to the therapy.

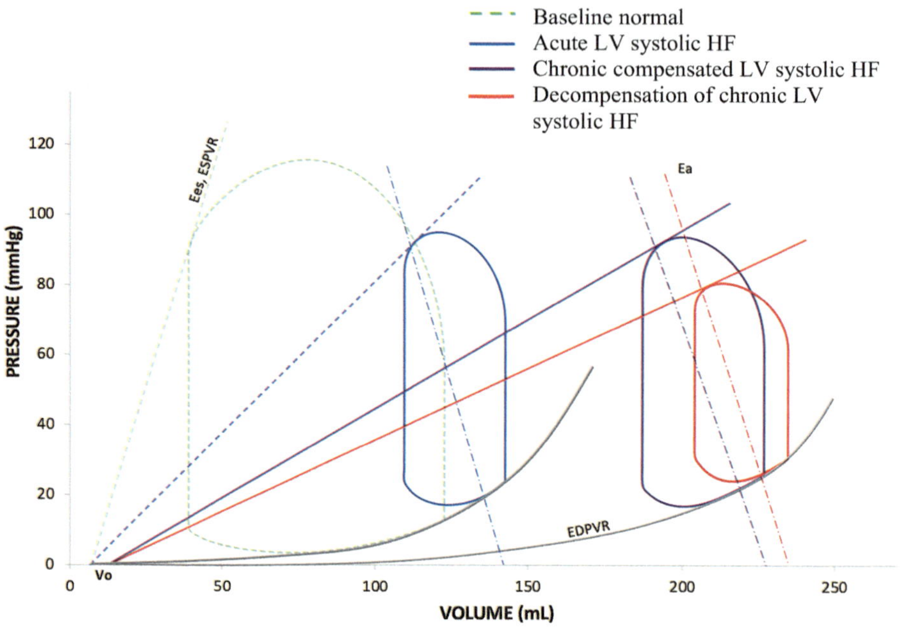

Fig. 9.2 *Decompensation of chronic LV systolic HF due to a decrease in LV contractility and neurohormonal activation*. LV Ees has decreased, and Ea has increased due to an increase in SVR and HR. The increase in Ea/Ees has caused the EF and SV to decrease further, the ESV to increase. Pes has decreased because despite the increase in Ea, Ees has decreased to a greater extent. The EDV has increased because of the increase in ESV plus an increase in systemic venous return. The latter is due to venoconstriction and an increase in total blood volume (fluid retention), each of which contribute to increasing the SBV and systemic venous return (see Chap. 5). The EDP has increased from an elevated baseline (22–30 mmHg), causing dyspnea and impaired oxygenation

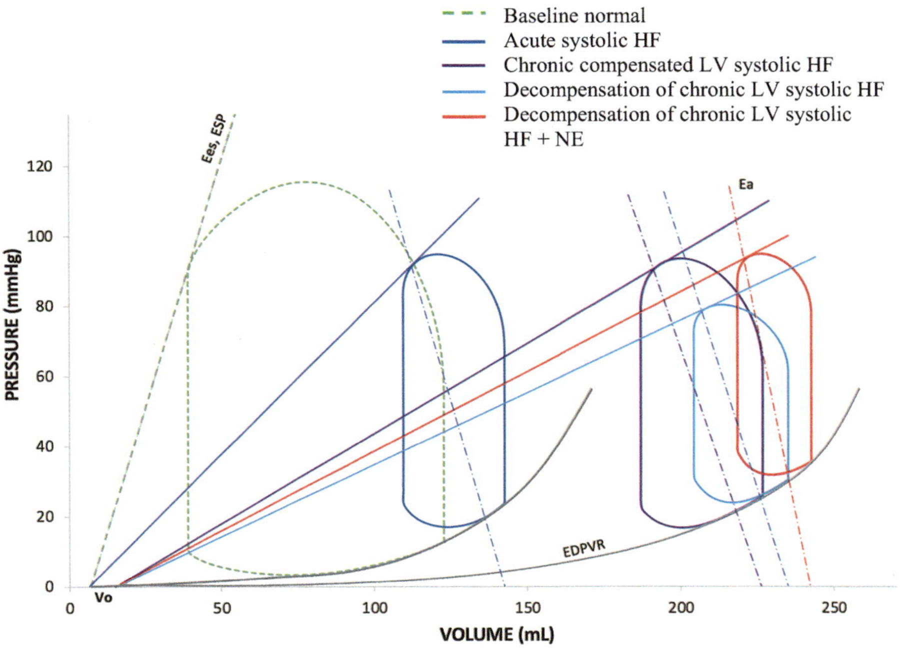

Fig. 9.3 *Inoconstrictor in decompensated chronic LV systolic HF.* The inoconstrictor NE has increased both Ea (SVR has increased considerably, as well as HR) and Ees. Because NE induces a greater increase in Ea than Ees, Ea/Ees and the extent of ventricular-arterial uncoupling have increased further. As a result, the EF and SV have decreased. The increase in both Ea and Ees increases Pes. Due to the increase in ESV and NE-induced venoconstriction and increase in SBV, the EDV and EDP have increased appreciably from an elevated baseline. Despite this, the CPP has increased as perfusion pressures have increased

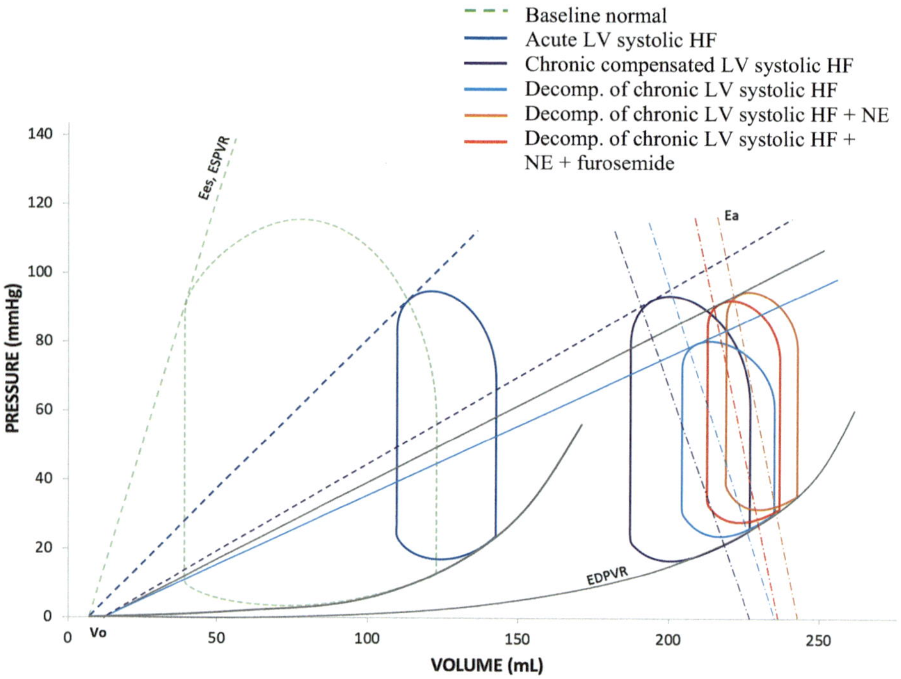

Fig. 9.4 *The inoconstrictor (NE) plus diuretic in decompensated chronic LV systolic HF*. These PVLs illustrate the sequential impact of the inoconstrictor NE plus the diuretic furosemide. Ea, Ees, and Ea/Ees remain unchanged. Due to furosemide induced venodilation and increase in venous capacitance and diuresis and decrease in total blood volume, the SBV and EDV decrease [24]. The modest decrease in LV EDV has significantly reduced the EDP because at large volumes operating stiffness is significantly elevated

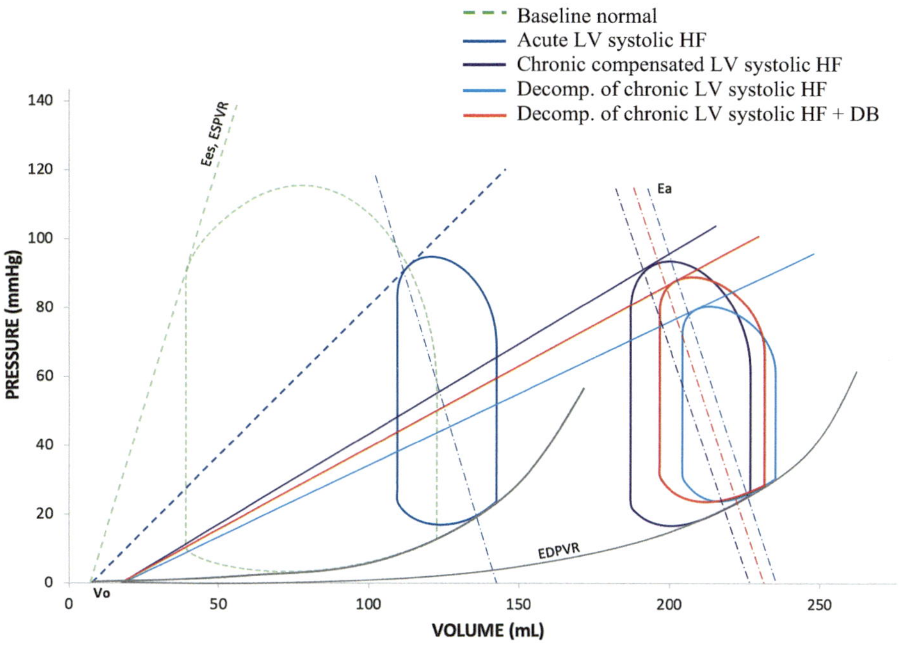

Fig. 9.5 *Inodilator in decompensated chronic LV systolic HF.* The inodilator DB has had little effect on Ea as a modest decrease in SVR has been offset by an increase in HR. DB was titrated to generate a similar increase in Ees as occurred with NE. Because Ea/Ees has decreased by 25%, the EF and SV have increased. And because Ees has increased while Ea remains unchanged, Pes, as well as mean and systolic BP, has increased, and perfusion pressures are adequate. Despite its vasodilatory properties, LV afterload has increased (systolic BP). The decrease in ESV coupled with DB-induced venodilation has decreased the SBV causing the EDV and EDP to decrease With similar increases in Ees and HR, mechanical efficiency (SW/PVA) was greater and myocardial VO_2 less with the inodilator than with the inoconstrictor due to the impact of each on Ea/Ees (see Chap. 2). For similar reasons, CO was greater (3.8 vs. 2.6 L/min) and the EDP less (28 vs. 38 mmHg) with the inodilator strategy. While the increase in aortic diastolic pressure was greater with the inoconstrictor NE, the CPP has increased to a similar degree with DB due to the significant difference in the effect of each agent on the EDP

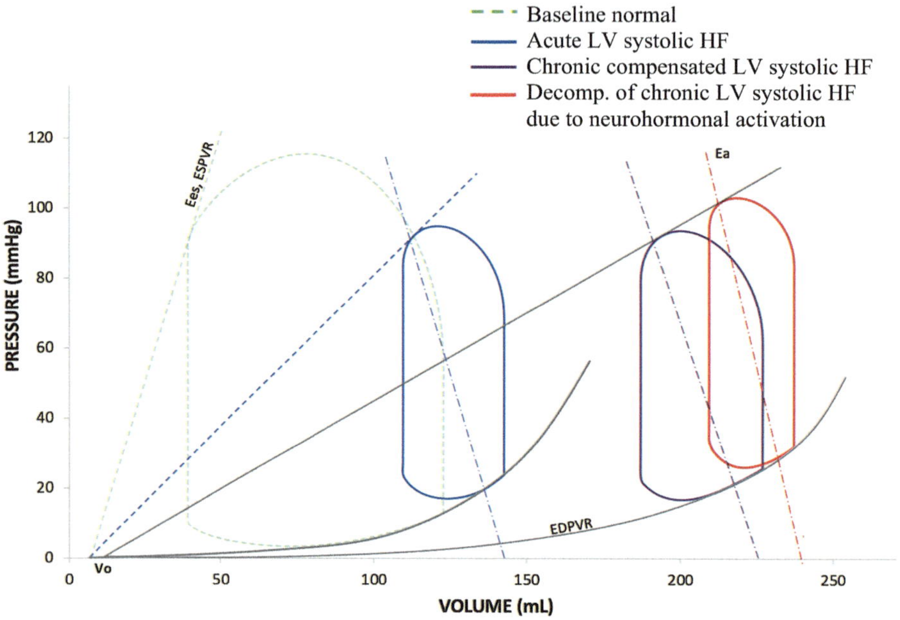

Fig. 9.6 *Decompensation of chronic LV systolic HF due to neurohormonal activation*. In contrast to the decompensation simulated in Figs. 9.2, 9.3, 9.4, and 9.5, where Ees decreased to a greater extent than Ea increased and thus aortic pressures decreased, decompensation here is the result of solely neurohormonal activation (SVR, HR, and SBV have increased). The isolated increase in Ea has increased Pes as well as mean and systolic pressures. The EF and SV have decreased; however, the worsening ventricular arterial uncoupling is due to the increase in Ea rather than a change in Ees

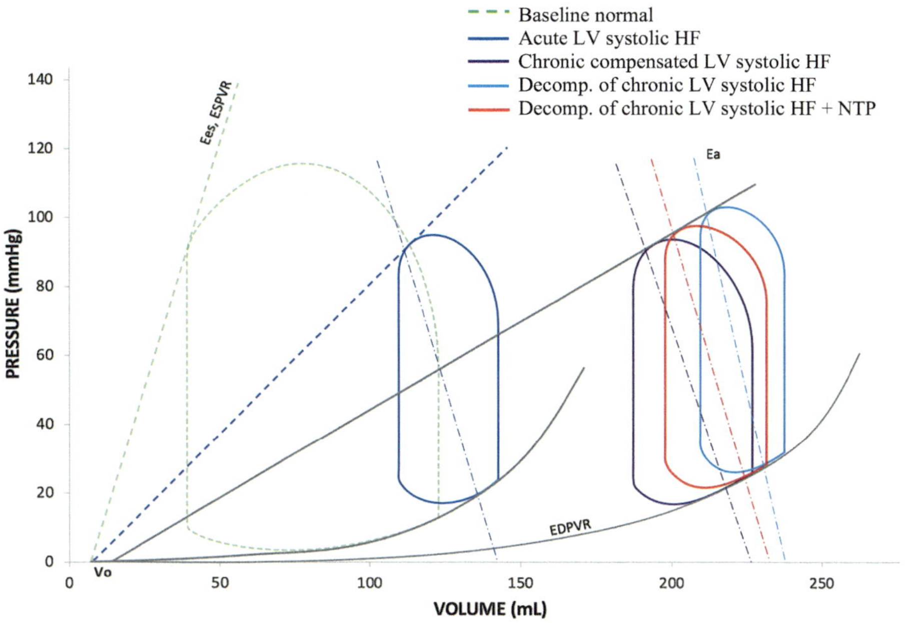

Fig. 9.7 *Vasodilator in decompensated chronic LV systolic HF due to neurohormonal activation.* The vasoactive agent NTP vasodilates arterial resistance and venous capacitance vessels. In this instance, NTP has returned hemodynamic parameters back toward baseline conditions. Ea and Ea/Ees have decreased, and the EF and SV have increased. The isolated decrease in Ea decreases the Pes. With NTP, the arterial load (Ea) and ventricular afterload (systolic BP) are reduced. Venodilation-induced decrease in SBV coupled with a decrease in ESV has significantly reduced the EDV and EDP. Myocardial VO_2 approaches baseline levels as ventricular loading conditions have improved (PVA is reduced) while contractility and HR are unchanged. The aortic diastolic pressure has decreased; however, the CPPs are similar because of the decrease in EDP

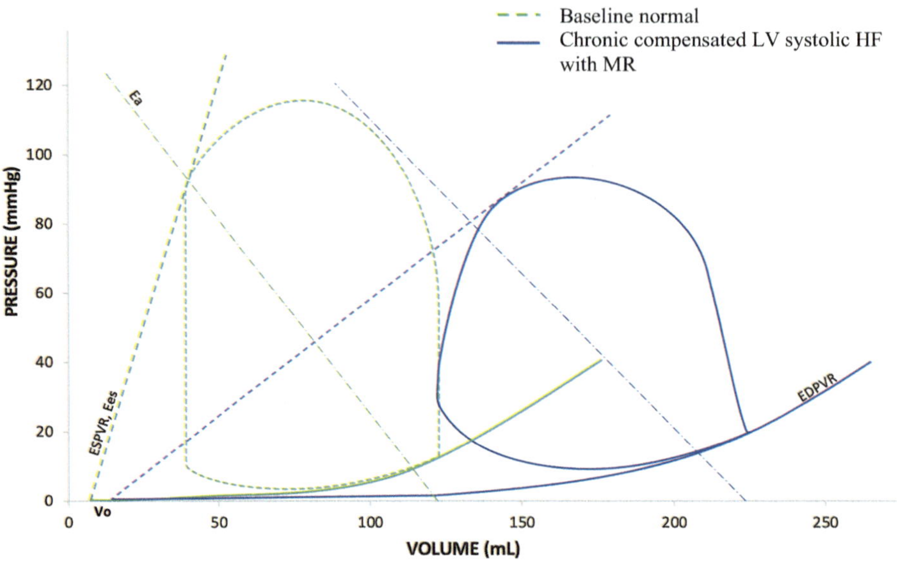

Fig. 9.8 *Chronic compensated LV systolic HF with functional MR*. This figure contrasts the PVL of a normal LV to the PVL of an LV which has undergone ventricular remodeling and marked chamber enlargement and the development of secondary or functional MR. MR is discussed in greater detail in Chap. 12. With MR, the isovolumic contraction phase of the cardiac cycle is absent. LV ejection starts with the regurgitant flow as soon as ventricular pressure rises above left atrial pressure. The isovolumic relaxation phase of the cardiac cycle is absent as well. Following aortic valve closure regurgitation continues as ventricular pressure is greater than left atrial pressure. Regurgitation reduces LV volume until LV pressure falls below left atrial pressure

In MR, the forward SV (not apparent in the PVL) or total SV (regurgitant plus forward volumes) may be used to determine Ea [25–28]. Ea based on the total SV ("Ea total"—depicted above) reflects the total afterload on the LV, both the arterial load and low impedance pathway provided by the left atrium. Ea based on the forward SV ("Ea forward") determines solely the arterial load. Because the EF is based on total ventricular afterload (Ea total/Ees), the EF in MR overestimates systolic function. In this instance, the EF in chronic systolic HF with secondary MR is only slightly less than the lower limit of normal because of the regurgitation

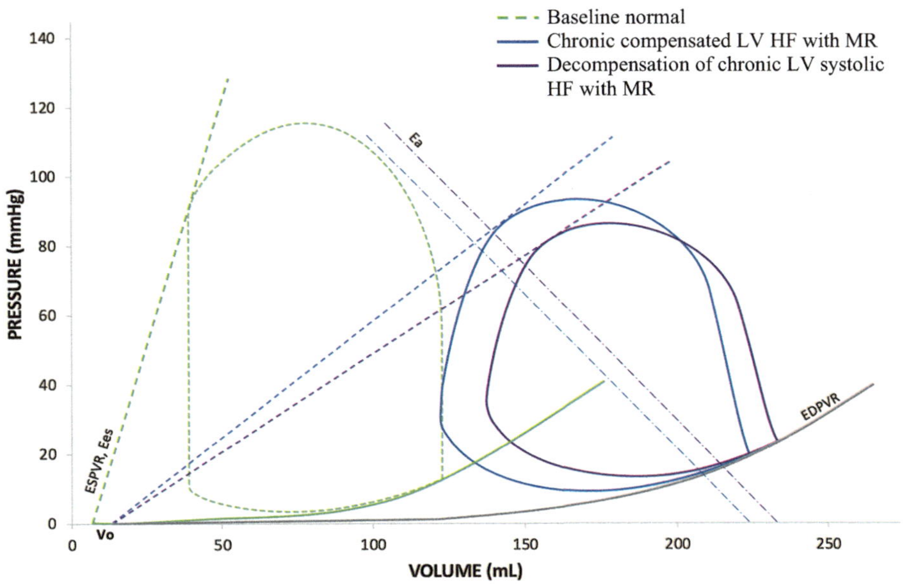

Fig. 9.9 *Decompensation of chronic LV systolic HF with functional MR.* These PVLs illustrate that the decompensation has resulted solely from a decrease in LV contractility. The degree of mitral incompetence has not changed nor has the arterial load (Ea forward); thus, Ea total (depicted above) has not changed. The increase in Ea total/Ees causes the EF and total SV to decrease. As a result, both forward and regurgitant volumes have decreased, and the RF is unchanged. The EDP has increased from an elevated baseline

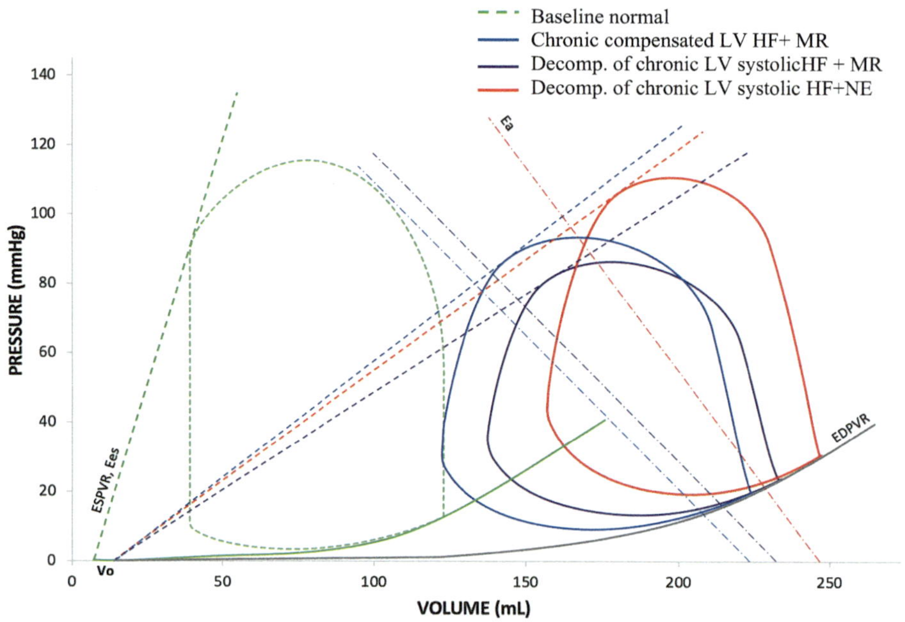

Fig. 9.10 *Inoconstrictor in decompensated chronic LV systolic HF with functional MR.* In this instance, the inoconstrictor NE has nearly restored contractility to its pre-decompensation level, while significantly increasing SVR, HR and thus Ea forward and Ea total. Because Ea total has increased to a greater extent than Ees, Ea total/Ees has increased, and as a result, the EF and total SV (~10%) have decreased. The forward SV has decreased by ~30% and the regurgitant volume and RF have increased, which coupled with the increase in ESV and NE-induced increase in SBV, have significantly increased the EDP (24–30 mmHg). Despite the increase in EDP, the CPP has increased due to the rise in aortic diastolic pressure

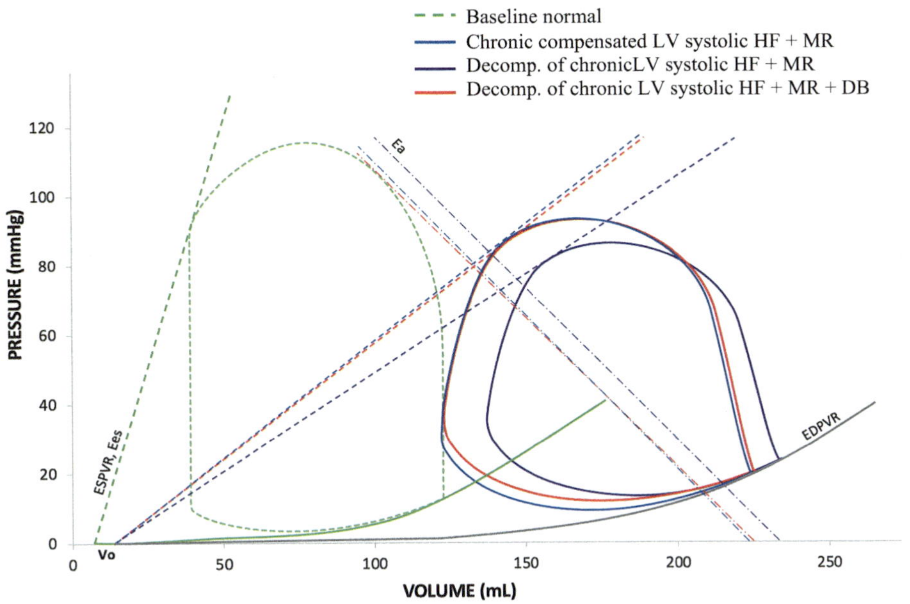

Fig. 9.11 *Inodilator in decompensated chronic LV systolic HF with functional MR.* In this instance, the inodilator DB was titrated to increase Ees to the same extent as occurred with NE. LV Ees has returned to baseline. DB has caused a modest decrease in SVR, which has been offset by an increase in HR. As a result, Ea forward and Ea total are unchanged. Ea total/Ees has returned to the pre-decompensation level, restoring the total SV and forward SV. The EDP and systemic pressures have also returned to pre-decompensation levels

With similar incremental changes in Ees and HR for the inoconstrictor and inodilator, the forward SV and CO are much greater (~35% and > 1.5 L/minute, respectively) and the EDP much less (20 vs. 30 mmHg) with the inodilator. The increase in perfusion pressure is far less than that seen for NE, however, with the decrease in LV EDP, the CPP has risen to >40 mmHg. Myocardial VO_2 was considerably less with the inodilator as the PVA was ~20% less

References

1. Fudim M, Kaye DM, Borlaug BA, et al. Venous tone and stressed blood volume in heart failure. J Am Coll Cardiol. 2022;79:1858–69.
2. Mann DL, Barger PM, Burkhoff D. Myocardial recovery and the failing heart. J Am Coll Cardiol. 2012;60:2465–72.
3. Gonzalez A, Ravassa S, Beaumont J, et al. New targets to treat structural remodeling of the myocardium. J Am Coll Cardiol. 2011;58:1833–43.
4. Cohn JN, Ferrari R, Sharpe N, et al. Cardiac remodeling—concepts and clinical implications: a consensus paper from an international forum on cardiac remodeling. J Am Coll Cardiol. 2000;35:569–82.
5. Furer A, Wessler J, Burkhoff D. Hemodynamics of cardiogenic shock. Interv Cardiol Clin. 2017;6:359–71.
6. Burkhoff D. Pressure-volume loops in clinical research. J Am Coll Cardiol. 2013;62:1173–6.
7. McMurray J. Systolic heart failure. N Engl J Med. 2010;362:228–338.

8. Hill JA, Olson EN. Cardiac plasticity. N Engl J Med. 2008;358:1370–80.
9. Enriquez-Sarano M, Loulmet DF, Burkhoff D. The conundrum of functional mitral regurgitation in chronic heart failure. J Am Coll Cardiol. 2008;51:487–9.
10. Pierard LA, Lancellotti P. The role of ischemic mitral regurgitation in the pathogenesis of acute pulmonary edema. N Engl J Med. 2004;351:1627–34.
11. Punnoose L, Burkhoff D, Cunningham L, et al. Functional mitral regurgitation: therapeutic strategies for a ventricular disease. J Card Fail. 2014;20:252–67.
12. Asgar AW, Mack MJ, Stone GW. Secondary mitral regurgitation in heart failure. J Am Coll Cardiol. 2015;65:1231–48.
13. Gaasch WH, Meyer TE. Secondary mitral regurgitation (part 1): volumetric quantification and analysis. Heart. 2018;104:634–8.
14. Uhley HN, Leeds SE, Sampson JJ, et al. Right duct lymph flow in experimental heart failure following acute elevation of left atrial pressure. Circ Res. 1967;20:306–10.
15. Kay JM, Edwards FR. Ultrastructure of the alveolar-capillary wall in mitral stenosis. J Pathol. 1973;III:239–45.
16. Assayag P, Benamer H, Aubry P, et al. Alteration of the alveolar-capillary membrane diffusing capacity in chronic left heart disease. Am J Cardiol. 1998;82:459–64.
17. Kingsbury MP, Huang W, Donnelly JL, et al. Structural remodeling of lungs in chronic heart failure. Basic Res Cardiol. 2003;98:295–303.
18. Laine GA, Allen SJ, Katz J, et al. Effect of systemic venous pressure elevation on lymph flow and lung edema formation. J Appl Physiol. 1986;61:1634–8.
19. Robertson HT. Gas exchange consequences of left heart failure. Compr Physiol. 2011;1:621–34.
20. Guazzi M, Naeije R. Pulmonary hypertension in heart failure. J Am Coll Cardiol. 2017;69:1718–34.
21. Van Diepen S, Katz JN, Albert NM, et al. Contemporary management of cardiogenic shock. A scientific statement from the American heart association. Circulation. 2017;136:e232–68.
22. Heidenreich PA, Bozkurt B, Aguilar D, et al. 2022 AHA/ACC/HFSA guideline for the management of heart failure: a report of the American College of Cardiology/American Heart Association Joint Committee on clinical practice guidelines. Circulation. 2022;145:e895–e1032.
23. Law YM, Lal AK, Chen S, et al. Diagnosis and management of myocarditis in children. A scientific statement from the American heart association. Circulation. 2021;144:e123–35.
24. Dikshit K, Vyden JK, Forrester JS, et al. Renal and extrarenal hemodynamic effects of furosemide in congestive heart failure after acute myocardial infarction. N Engl J Med. 1973;288:1087–90.
25. Osuga T, Morita T, Sasaki N, et al. Prognostic value of left ventricular-arterial coupling estimated using echocardiography in dogs with myxomatous mitral valve disease. J Vet Intern Med. 2021;35:2607–15.
26. Starling MR. Left ventricular pump efficiency in long-term mitral regurgitation assessed by means of left ventricular-arterial coupling relations. Am Heart J. 1994;127:1324–35.
27. Imasaka K, Tayama E, Tomita Y. Left ventricular performance early after repair for posterior mitral leaflet prolapse: chordal replacement versus leaflet resection. J Thorac Cardiovasc Surg. 2015;150:538–45.
28. Lavall D, Reil J-C, Schmitz L, et al. Early hemodynamic improvement after percutaneous mitral valve repair evaluated by noninvasive pressure-volume analysis. J Am Soc Echocardiogr. 2016;29:888–98.

Chapter 10
Severe Sepsis and Septic Shock

Cameron Dezfulian, Hernando Gomez, and Michael R. Pinsky

Severe sepsis is clinically challenging to manage in part because of its heterogenic presentation and evolution. The nature of the invading organism, the host response, and the underlying cardiovascular function and comorbidities all converge to produce a wide spectrum of disease and hemodynamic phenotypes on presentation [1–7]. The ensuing inflammatory response may affect every aspect of the circulation [7–17], including alterations in vasomotor tone of the pulmonary and systemic arterial resistance and venous capacitance vessels [7–10], biventricular diastolic (impaired relaxation and increased ventricular stiffness), and systolic function [11–17].

Further confounding the management of severe sepsis is the varied response to therapies and the evolution of the disease including the development of multi-organ system injury and dysfunction. Complex cardio-renal and cardio-pulmonary interactions, for example, further challenge the clinician in determining the physiologic substrate and optimal therapies. The development of acute lung injury/acute respiratory distress syndrome (ARDS) and the provision of positive pressure ventilation may precipitate cor pulmonale (discussed in Chap. 15), which has an incidence ranging from 30 to 35% in children and adults and is associated with mortality [18, 19].

In the setting of such clinical heterogeneity, an algorithmic approach to the resuscitation of severe sepsis/septic shock as suggested by consensus-driven guidelines can be problematic [20–23]. Prior examinations of adult patients with septic shock [6] demonstrated that the hemodynamic response of patients (mean arterial

C. Dezfulian (✉)
Baylor College of Medicine, Texas Children's Hospital, Houston, TX, USA
e-mail: cxdezful@texaschildrens.org

H. Gomez · M. R. Pinsky
University of Pittsburgh School of Medicine, Pittsburgh, PA, USA
e-mail: gomezh@upmc.edu; pinsky@pitt.edu

R. A. Bronicki et al. (eds.), *Simulation in Cardiovascular Critical Care Medicine*, https://doi.org/10.1007/978-3-031-63557-1_10

pressure and cardiac index) to volume resuscitation was highly variable. In those patients with persistent hypotension or low cardiac index following volume loading, the response to inoconstrictors and inodilators also varied.

The variations in hemodynamic phenotypes on presentation and response to therapies precludes a simple formulaic approach to the treatment of severe sepsis. Limiting the characterization of cardiovascular dysfunction to simply hypotension despite fluid resuscitation, and the nonselective use of vasoactive therapy, fails to address the pathophysiologic processes responsible for cardiovascular dysfunction. Different initial physiologic states respond differently to defined clinical interventions. Thus, establishing a baseline hemodynamic phenotype and the application of known cardiovascular principles provides a framework from which to predict the response of the circulation to interventions and to tailor a more personalized therapy accordingly.

We used the Harvi cardiovascular simulator (PVLoops, LLC) to illustrate the impact of the consensus-generated algorithmic resuscitation-based guidelines in an adolescent/young adult patient presenting with a spectrum of sepsis-induced hemodynamic phenotypes (Figs. 10.1a, 10.1b, 10.1c, 10.2a, 10.2b, 10.2c, 10.2d, 10.2e, 10.3a, 10.3b, 10.3c, and 10.3d). The most recent consensus-generated guidelines for the treatment of severe sepsis recommends 40–60 ml/kg over the first hour for children [20], while the recommendation for adults is at least 30 ml/kg over the first three hours [21]. Although these recommendations have been downgraded from strong to weak, they still dominate the clinical approach to early sepsis resuscitation. If hypotension or inadequate perfusion persists despite this initial fluid resuscitation, vasoactive therapy is recommended. Recently published consensus-generated guidelines vary on which vasoactive agents to use—vasopressor, inoconstrictor, or inodilator—and their sequence [20–23]. For these reasons, we have simulated the impact of fluid administration followed by the impact of either an inoconstrictor, vasopressor, or inodilator in patients with varying hemodynamic phenotypes of severe sepsis. The emphasis here is on the *effects* of each agent on the circulation and in turn pressure and flow rather than the *agent or class of agent* selected. The changes in magnitude of the hemodynamic parameters may vary depending on the host response to therapy. We have limited the exercise to evaluating the impact of disease and therapy on the systemic circulation and left ventricle.

The decrease in SV was less with NE than AVP. The increase in Ea with each agent was similar however the increase in Ees with NE partially offset the increase in Ea. Thus, the increase in Ea/Ees and resulting decrease in EF and SV was less with NE than AVP.

When comparing the inoconstrictor to inodilator strategy, SV, CO and DO_2 are greater (by 10%, 600 ml/min, 110 ml/min, respectively) and the EDP less (25 vs 21 mmHg) with the inodilator. The PVA is considerably less and mechanical efficiency greater with the inodilator. However, because of a greater increase in HR with DB, myocardial VO_2 was similar.

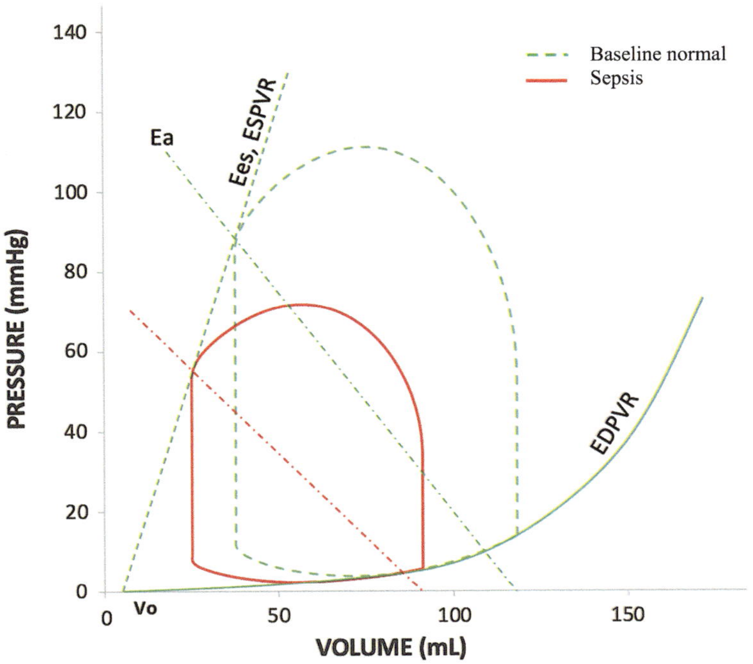

Fig. 10.1a *Severe sepsis characterized by vasoplegia.* These LV PVLs illustrate findings consistent with the development of vasoplegia in an adolescent patient. LV Ees is unaffected, while Ea, EDV, SV, and arterial pressures have decreased, which is consistent with the onset of severe sepsis characterized by vasoplegia (significant decrease in tone in the systemic arterial resistance and venous capacitance vessels). In this instance, reduced Ea results from a significant decrease in SVR despite a significant increase in HR. The reduced arterial load (Ea) and decrease in Ea/Ees cause the EF to increase (68–76%); however, the SV has decreased due to a significant decrease in EDV, which results from tachycardia and reduced filling time and a decrease in the systemic venous return. The latter results from venodilation and an increase in the unstressed blood volume, and vascular leak and decrease in total blood volume, each of which contribute to a significant decrease in SBV and in turn systemic venous return (see Chap. 5). The perfusion pressures are critically low (mean BP and CPP are 50 and 28 mmHg, respectively). Because of the tachycardia, CO and DO_2 have risen by some 25% and the oxygen extraction is less than normal

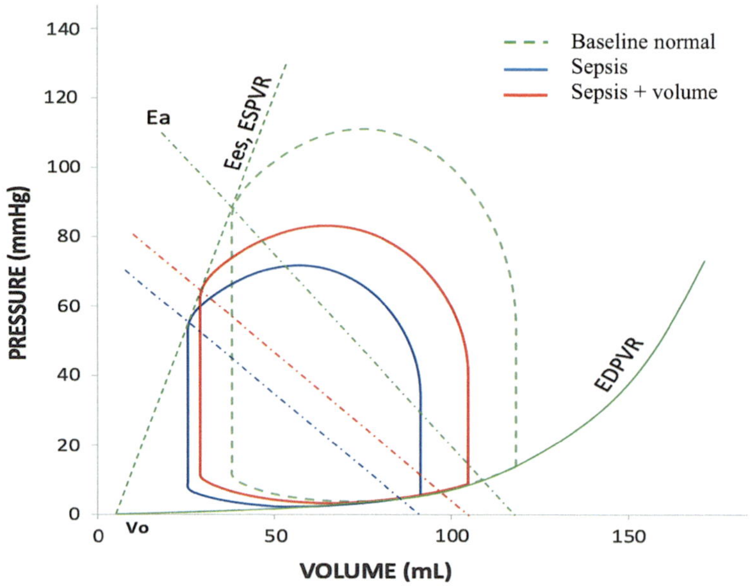

Fig. 10.1b *Severe sepsis with vasoplegia treated with intravascular volume.* These PVLs illustrate the effects of intravascular volume (40 cc/kg) and increase in total blood volume, SBV, and ultimately LV EDV. The SV and arterial pressures increase. Ees and Ea are unaffected by changes in preload (EDV). Despite the increase in SV, the patient remains hypotensive with inadequate perfusion pressures (mean BP 58 mmHg, CPP 31 mm Hg) due to persistently low systemic arterial and venous tone

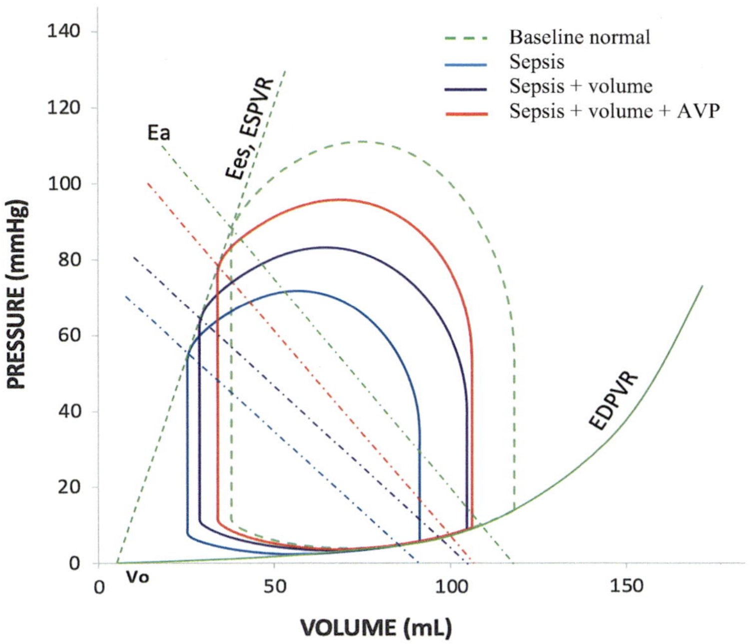

Fig. 10.1c *Severe sepsis with vasoplegia treated with intravascular volume and a vasopressor.* The vasopressor AVP increases SVR and Ea without effecting Ees, thus Ea/Ees increases, the EF and SV decrease, while the perfusion pressures (CPP, mean BP) rise above the minimum recommended pressures of 45 and 65 mmHg, respectively, for an adult. The HR is unaffected, and CO and DO_2 decrease but remain greater than baseline normal

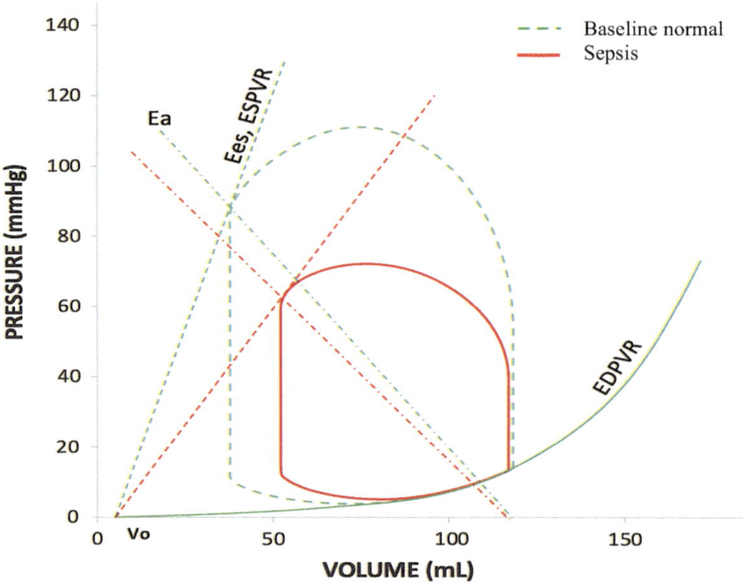

Fig. 10.2a *Severe sepsis with decrease LV contractility and diminished vascular tone.* These LV PVLs illustrate decrease function and vasomotor tone in an adolescent patient with sepsis. LV contractility and Ees are significantly reduced, while the decrease in SVR and Ea is less severe. The EF remains in the normal range at 55% despite the significant decrease in contractility because the decrease in Ees is partially offset by the decrease in Ea. The increase in Ea/Ees causes the SV to decrease, the ESV to increase. The perfusion pressures are inadequate due to the decrease in both Ea and Ees. Notably, despite the significant decrease in LV systolic function, the EDV and EDP are normal, because of the concurrent decrease in venomotor tone, SBV, and systemic venous return

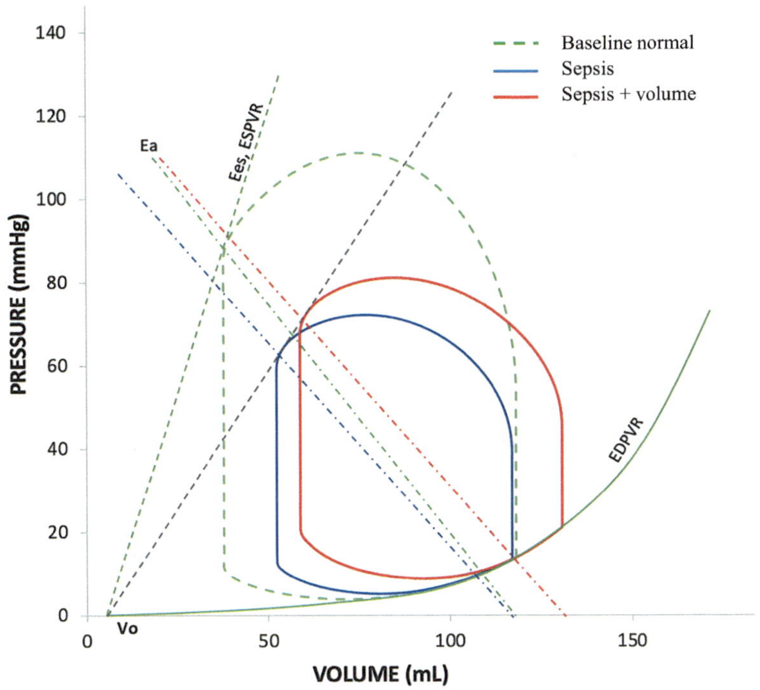

Fig. 10.2b *Severe sepsis with decrease LV contractility and diminished vascular tone treated with intravascular volume.* Intravascular volume (40 cc/kg) increases the SV and arterial pressures. Despite the increase in aortic pressure, the CPP has decreased further, as the EDP has risen to a greater extent than the aortic diastolic pressure. The EF remains unchanged (55%) and in the range of normal as Ea/Ees is unaffected by intravascular volume. Persistent ventricular arterial uncoupling and the increase in TBV and SBV increase the EDV and EDP, resulting in cardiogenic pulmonary edema. If this had occurred in the setting of acute lung injury/acute respiratory distress syndrome (ARDS), the rate and extent of extravascular lung water formation would be much greater

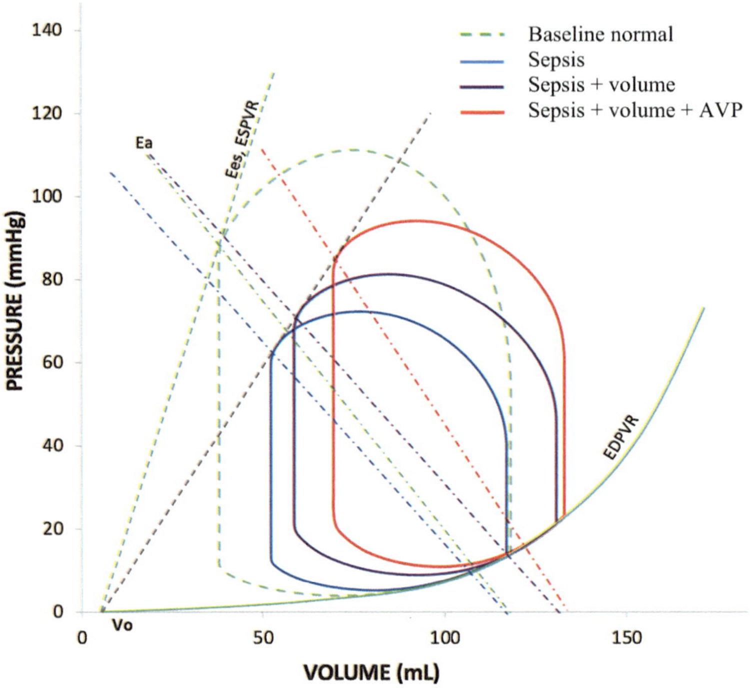

Fig. 10.2c *Severe sepsis with decrease LV contractility and diminished vascular tone treated with intravascular volume and a vasopressor.* These PVLs illustrate the effect of intravascular volume expansion followed by the addition of the vasopressor AVP. AVP increases SVR, restoring a near normal Ea. Thus, Ea/Ees and the extent of ventricular arterial uncoupling worsens, causing the EF and SV to decrease further (55–47% and 72–64 ml, respectively). The increase in ESV coupled with AVP-induced venoconstriction increases the SBV and in turn systemic venous return, the LV EDV and LV EDP, worsening the degree of cardiogenic pulmonary edema. The increase in Ea increases the Pes as well as mean and systolic pressures; however, the CPP is marginal. By normalizing ventricular loading conditions, the extent of systolic dysfunction becomes increasingly more apparent based on the EF and significantly elevated LV EDV and EDP

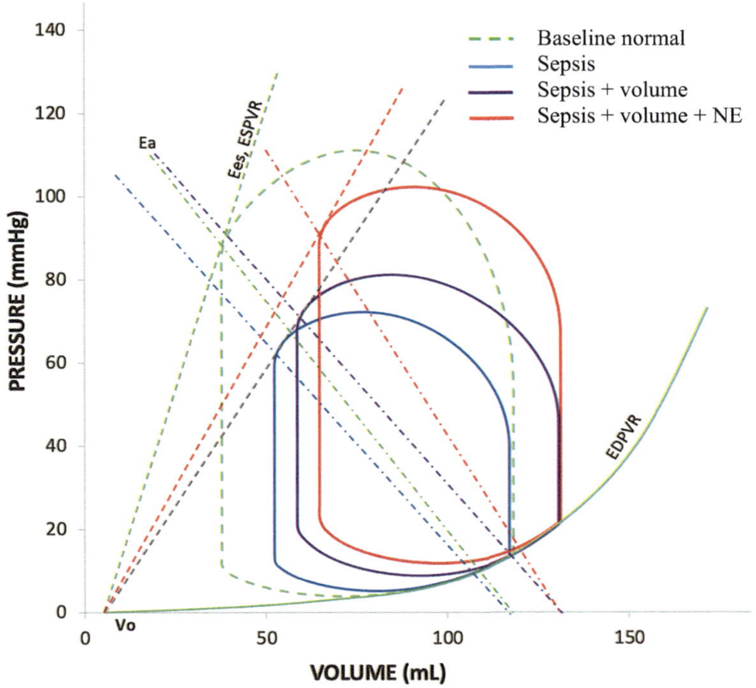

Fig. 10.2d *Severe sepsis with decrease contractility and diminished vascular tone treated with intravascular volume and an inoconstrictor.* These PVLs illustrate the effect of volume expansion followed by the administration of the inoconstrictor NE. NE has increased Ea (SVR and less so HR) to a somewhat greater extent than Ees, causing the Ea/Ees to increase, the EF and SV to decrease. The increase in ESV coupled with NE-induced venoconstriction further increases the SBV, EDV, and EDP. The increase in Ea and Ees increases Pes as well as mean and systolic pressures. There is little change in CO and DO_2 as the decrease in SV is offset by an increase in HR

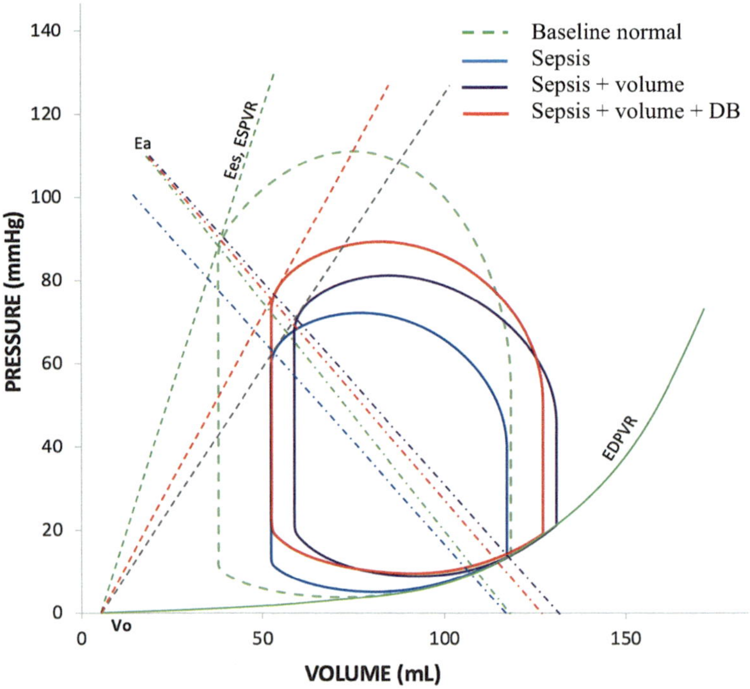

Fig. 10.2e *Severe sepsis with decrease contractility and diminished vascular tone treated with intravascular volume and an inodilator.* These PVLs illustrate the effect of volume expansion followed by the administration of the inodilator DB. DB has increased Ees (titrated such that the increase in Ees was similar to that induced by NE) with little change in Ea (SVR decreases but it is offset by an increase in HR). The decrease in Ea/Ees increases the EF and SV. The increase in Ees with little change in Ea increases the Pes as well as mean and systolic pressures. The perfusion pressures now exceed the minimum recommended values for an adolescent/adult (mean BP > 65 and systolic BP > 90 mmHg, respectively). The EDP has decreased due to the decrease in ESV coupled with DB-induced venodilation and decrease in SBV

Comparing NE to DB, with similar effects on Ees, CO is considerably greater (800 ml/min) and EDP lower (22 vs. 17 mmHg) with the inodilator strategy. The PVA is considerably less (some 20%) and mechanical efficiency greater with the inodilator; however, because of a greater increase in HR with DB, the difference in myocardial VO_2 is less

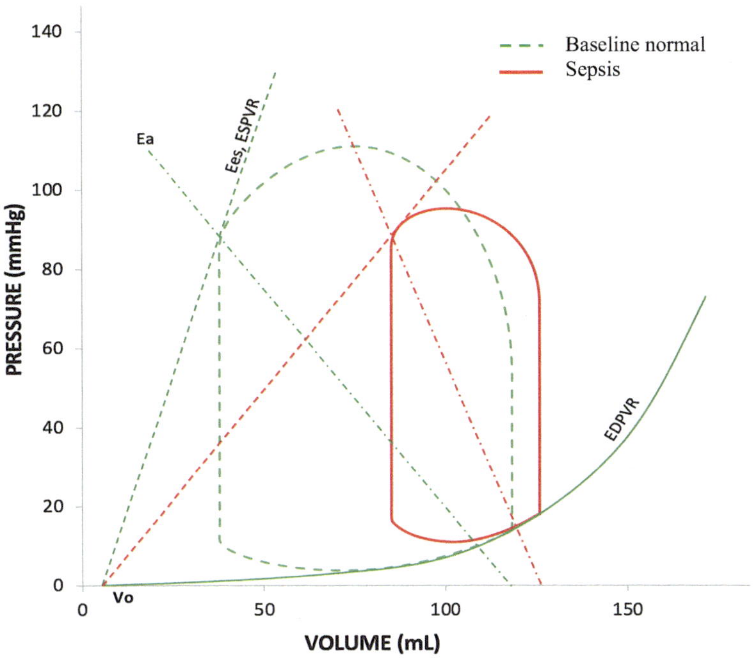

Fig. 10.3a *Severe sepsis with decrease contractility and elevated vascular tone.* These PVLs illustrate findings consistent with the onset of severe sepsis in an adolescent patient characterized by decreased LV contractility (Ees), increase in Ea (increase in SVR and HR), and elevated ESV and EDV. This hemodynamic phenotype of severe sepsis is consistent with cardiogenic shock where contractility is acutely and severely depressed and neurohormonal activation has increased systemic arterial and venomotor tone. Ea/Ees is significantly elevated, resulting in a significantly reduced EF (32%) and SV (~50% decrease). The Pes remains unchanged as the decrease in Ees is offset by the increase in Ea. The significant decrement in SV narrows the pulse pressure with a low systolic BP, elevated diastolic BP, and preserved mean BP. The increase in ESV coupled with an increase in venomotor tone and SBV increase the EDV and EDP, resulting in cardiogenic pulmonary edema. As in the previous sepsis simulation, if this had occurred in the setting of acute lung injury/acute respiratory distress syndrome (ARDS), the rate and extent of extravascular lung water formation would be much greater

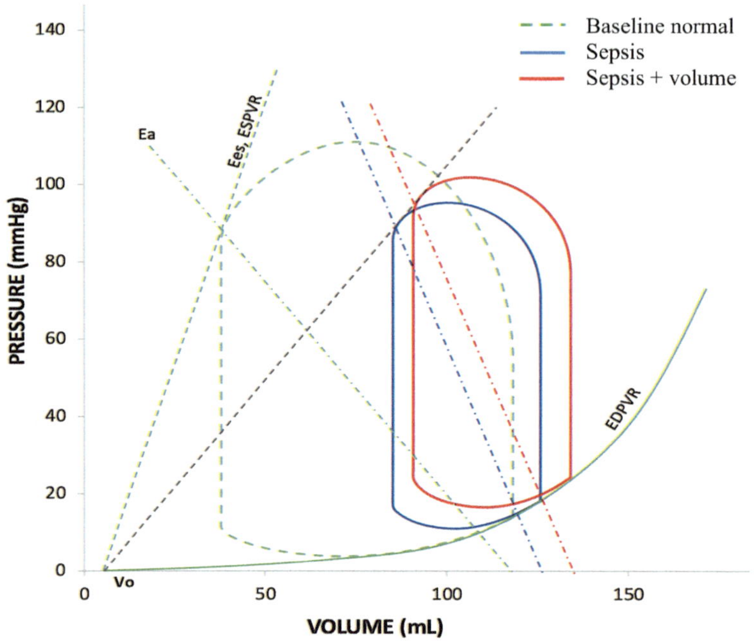

Fig. 10.3b *Severe sepsis with decrease contractility and elevated vascular tone treated with intravascular volume.* Intravascular volume (40 cc/kg) has a modest impact on SV and BP; however, the increase in EDV and EDP worsens the cardiogenic pulmonary edema. While the resulting increase in EDV was limited, the EDP increased considerably due to the increase in operating stiffness at large volumes

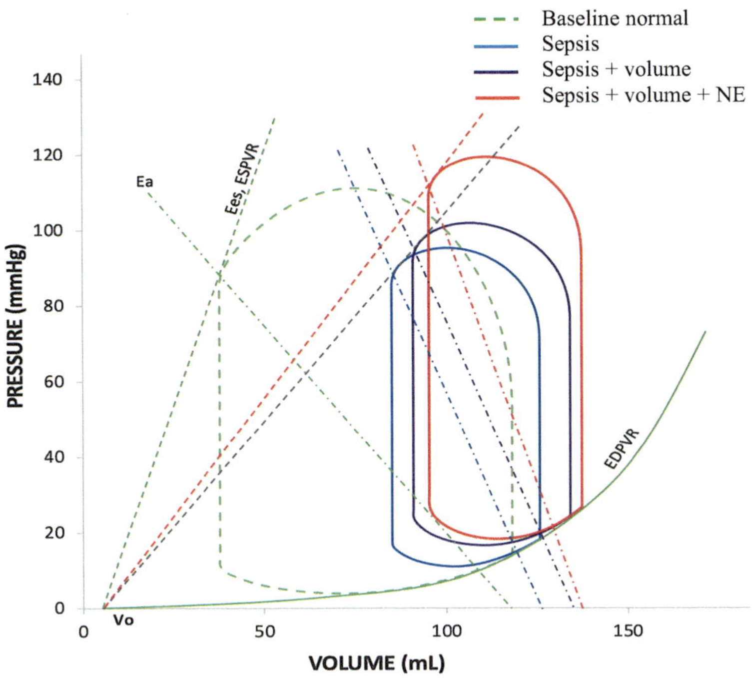

Fig. 10.3c *Severe sepsis with decrease contractility and elevated vascular tone treated with intravascular volume and an inoconstrictor.* These PVLs illustrate the impact of volume resuscitation followed by the initiation of the inoconstrictor NE. In this instance, NE increases Ea (SVR and HR) to a similar degree as Ees, thus the EF and SV are unchanged. Because of the increase in Ea and Ees, the Pes as well as mean and systolic pressures rise significantly. The EDP increases further due to a venoconstriction-induced increase in SBV

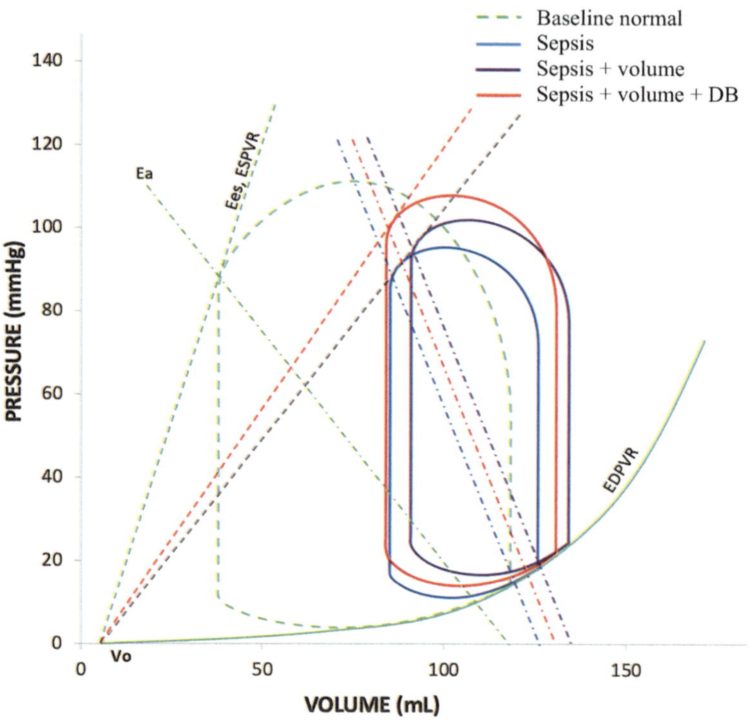

Fig. 10.3d *Severe sepsis with decrease contractility and elevated vascular tone treated with intravascular volume and an inodilator.* These PVLs illustrate the impact of volume resuscitation followed by the inodilator DB. In this instance, DB was titrated such that Ees increased to a similar extent as that induced by NE. Ea remains unchanged, as the decrease in SVR is offset by an increase in HR. The decrease in Ea/Ees increases the EF and SV and decreases the ESV. The increase in Ees without a change in Ea increases the Pes as well as mean and systolic pressures. Despite its vasodilatory effect, the systolic BP has increased and so too has LV afterload. The EDP decreases because of a decrease in ESV and DB-induced venodilation and decrease in SBV

References

1. Ceneviva G, Paschall A, Maffei F, et al. Hemodynamic support in fluid-refractory pediatric septic shock. Pediatrics. 1998;102:e19.
2. Parker MM, Shelhamer JH, Natanson C, et al. Serial cardiovascular variables in survivors and nonsurvivors of human septic shock: heart rate as an early predictor of prognosis. Crit Care Med. 1987;15:923–9.
3. Mercier J-C, Beaufils F, Hartmann J-F, et al. Hemodynamic patterns of meningococcal shock in children. Crit Care Med. 1988;16:27–33.
4. Carvaita S, Baratto C, Di Marco F, et al. Haemodynamic characteristics of COVID-19 patients with acute respiratory distress syndrome requiring mechanical ventilation. An invasive assessment using right heart catheterization. Eur J Heart Fail. 2020;22:2228–37.
5. Pollack MM, Fields AI, Ruttimann UE. Sequential cardiopulmonary variables of infants and children in septic shock. Crit Care Med. 1984;12:554–9.

6. Guarracino F, Bertini P, Pinsky MR. Cardiovascular determinants of resuscitation from sepsis and septic shock. Crit Care. 2019;22:118.
7. Vieillard-Baron A, Prin S, Chergui K, et al. Hemodynamic instability in sepsis. Am J Respir Crit Care Med. 2003;168:1270–6.
8. Perel A. Bench-to-bedside review: the initial hemodynamic resuscitation of the septic patient according to surviving sepsis campaign guideline—does one size fit all? Crit Care. 2008;12:223.
9. Guarracino F, Baldassarri R, Pinsky MR. Ventriculo-arterial decoupling in acutely altered hemodynamic states. Crit Care. 2013;17(2):213.
10. Guarracino F, Ferro B, Morelli A, et al. Ventriculoarterial decoupling in human septic shock. Crit Care. 2014;18(2):R80.
11. Werdan K, Müller-Werdan U. Elucidating molecular mechanisms of septic cardiomyopathy--the cardiomyocyte model. Mol Cell Biochem. 1996;163:291–303.
12. Martin L, Derwall M, Al Zoubi S, et al. The septic heart. Chest. 2019;155:427–37.
13. Beesley SJ, Weber G, Sarge T, et al. Septic cardiomyopathy. Crit Care Med. 2018;46:625–34.
14. Nishio R, Sasayama S, Matsumori A. Left ventricular pressure-volume relationship in a murine model of congestive heart failure due to acute viral myocarditis. J Am Coll Cardiol. 2002;40:1506–14.
15. Chagnon F, Bentourkia M, Lecomte R, et al. Endotoxin-induced heart dysfunction in rats: assessment of myocardial perfusion and permeability and the role of fluid resuscitation. Crit Care Med. 2006;34:127–33.
16. Yu P, Boughner DR, Sibbbald WJ, et al. Myocardial collagen changes and edema in rats with hyperdynamic sepsis. Crit Care Med. 1997;25:657–62.
17. Sanfilippo F, Corredor C, Arcadipane A, et al. Tissue Doppler assessment of diastolic function and relationship with mortality in critically ill septic patients: a systematic review and meta-analysis. Br J Anaesth. 2017;119:583–94.
18. Dessap A, Boissier F, Charron C, et al. Acute cor pulmonale during protective ventilation for acute respiratory distress syndrome: prevalence, predictors, and clinical impact. Intensive Care Med. 2016;42:862–70.
19. Himebauch AS, Yehya N, Wang Y, et al. Early right ventricular systolic dysfunction and pulmonary hypertension are associated with worse outcomes in pediatric acute respiratory distress syndrome. Crit Care Med. 2018;46:e1055–62.
20. Weiss SL, Peters MJ, Alhazzani W, et al. Surviving sepsis campaign international guidelines for the management of septic shock and sepsis-associated organ dysfunction in children. Pediatr Crit Care Med. 2020;21:e52–e106.
21. Evans L, Rhodes A, Alhazzani W, et al. Executive summary: surviving sepsis campaign: international guidelines for the management of sepsis and septic shock 2021. Crit Care Med. 2021;49:1974–82.
22. Levy MM, Evans LE, Rhodes A. The surviving sepsis campaign bundle: 2018 update. Intensive Care Med. 2018;44:925–8.
23. Davis AL, Carcillo JA, Aneja RK, et al. American College of Critical Care Medicine clinical practice parameters for hemodynamic support of pediatric and neonatal septic shock. Crit Care Med. 2017;45:1061–93.

Chapter 11
Mechanical Circulatory Support

Sebastian C. Tume, Ronald A. Bronicki, and Daniel Burkhoff

For patients with circulatory insufficiency, pharmacological therapies alone may not restore and maintain adequate myocardial and systemic oxygen delivery, in which case an acute mechanical circulatory support (AMCS) device is indicated. These devices may be deployed as a bridge to recovery, decision, or long-term support device. The optimal selection of an AMCS device and the timing of its placement remain unknown, and significant practice variability exists.

There are several AMCS devices that may be deployed. Each device may be distinguished by the characteristics of the pump, the size and configuration of the cannula(e) and whether they are placed percutaneously or surgically, the amount of flow it can provide, and whether it can support either or both ventricles and gas exchange [1–5]. The selection of a device is also contingent upon the age and size of the patient, right ventricular contractility and pulmonary arterial load and the extent of right ventricular-pulmonary artery uncoupling, valvular function, rhythm, and respiratory function. All devices to varying degrees improve cardiac output and blood pressure, but they each have specific features that result in different hemodynamic effects, particularly as it relates to their ability to unload the left ventricle.

AMCS devices include the intra-aortic balloon pump (IABP); a right or left atrial to pulmonary artery or aorta assist device (TandemHeart, CardiacAssist, Pittsburgh, PA); a right or left ventricular to pulmonary artery or aorta assist device (Impella, Abiomed, Danvers, MA); and venoarterial extracorporeal membrane oxygenation (VA ECMO) [1–5].

S. C. Tume · R. A. Bronicki (✉)
Baylor College of Medicine, Texas Children's Hospital, Houston, TX, USA
e-mail: sctume@texaschildrens.org; rxbronic@texaschildrens.org

D. Burkhoff
Cardiovascular Research Foundation, New York, NY, USA
e-mail: dburkhoff@crf.org

R. A. Bronicki et al. (eds.), *Simulation in Cardiovascular Critical Care Medicine*, https://doi.org/10.1007/978-3-031-63557-1_11

The goal of an AMCS device is not only to generate an adequate blood pressure and blood flow but also to optimize myocardial protection and preservation while minimizing injury to the lung.

A significant and acute rise in left atrial and pulmonary microvascular hydrostatic pressure from a normal or elevated baseline leads to hydrostatic pulmonary edema. When capillary stress rises to sufficient levels, frank disruptions may develop in the alveolar-blood barrier, a condition known as stress failure [6–9]. When this occurs, there is considerable overlap in the pathophysiology between permeability and hydrostatic pulmonary edema [6–9], which leads to fulminant pulmonary edema. The marked increase in vascular permeability also allows for the extravasation of serum proteins into alveoli, which impairs surfactant activity and increases alveolar surface tension forces and the propensity for alveolar collapse [7]. In these patients, an important goal of AMCS is to reduce left atrial pressure.

Myocardial protection and preservation are addressed by optimizing left ventricular loading conditions and in turn the relationship between myocardial oxygen consumption and delivery (energetics) [3, 4, 10, 11]. There may be additional benefits related to left ventricular decompression and reductions in mechanical stress separate from its impact on myocardial energetics [3, 4, 10–13].

With significantly reduced left ventricular diastolic volume and pressure and thus peak left ventricular systolic pressure, the ventricular pressure volume loop shifts down and to the left, indicative of a marked reduction in the left ventricular pressure volume area and myocardial oxygen consumption (see Chaps. 2 and 4). At the same time, by reducing elevated left ventricular diastolic volume and pressure, myocardial perfusion improves.

For these reasons, an important priority in patients on AMCS is to determine the extent of left ventricular loading. Echocardiography is invaluable for determining left ventricular dimensions and the degree of left ventricular filling and whether the aortic valve is opening. Because left ventricular stiffness and the effective compliance of the left ventricle are unknown, left ventricular chamber size may not be an accurate indicator of the left ventricular diastolic pressure. Sufficient unloading of the left ventricle is reflected in a marked reduction in left ventricular end diastolic volume and pressure, such that the pressure-generating ability of the left ventricle is markedly reduced.

There are several strategies for unloading the left ventricle. Each strategy has its advantages, disadvantages, and varying degrees of efficacy. In contrast to the other ACMS devices, VA ECMO does not decompress the left ventricle [3–5, 10, 11]. To the extent that left ventricle remains volume and pressure loaded, and with the notion that the myocardium is recoverable, there is considerable debate as to how aggressively to pursue left ventricular unloading in patients supported with VA ECMO, given the absence of definitive data on the benefit of decompression on limiting the extent of myocardial injury and optimizing myocardial preservation [10–21].

In the following simulations of acute left ventricular systolic heart failure and cardiogenic shock, the degree of circulatory support and left ventricular unloading provided by each device are illustrated (Figs. 11.1, 11.2, 11.3, 11.4, 11.5, 11.6, 11.7, 11.8, 11.9, and 11.10). Additional pharmacologic strategies may be used to unload the left ventricle such as diuretics and vasodilators of venous capacitance and arterial resistance vessels. For all the simulations, the baseline hemodynamic parameters are the same: significantly decreased LV contractility and significantly increased arterial load, stressed blood volume, and heart rate.

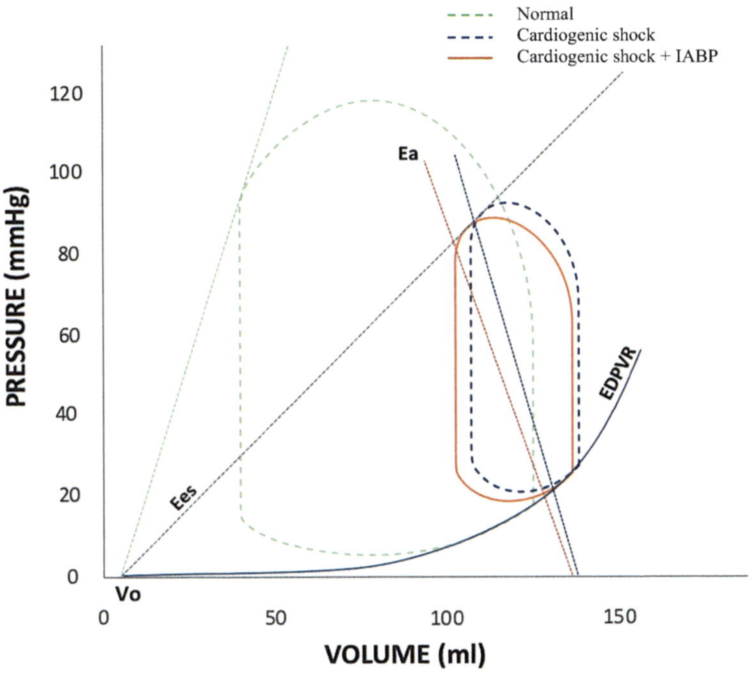

Fig. 11.1 *Cardiogenic shock plus intra-aortic balloon pump (IABP).* These PVLs illustrate the degree of circulatory support and LV unloading provided by an IABP. The IABP provides synchronized counterpulsation with inflation of the balloon during diastole, augmenting coronary perfusion, and deflation of the balloon during systole, reducing effective afterload. Patients must have some level of LV function and rhythm stability. The IABP provides limited enhancement of SV and CPP. The PVL is shifted down and to the left, indicative of a decrease in the PVA and myocardial VO_2. The degree to which the LV is unloaded is minimal

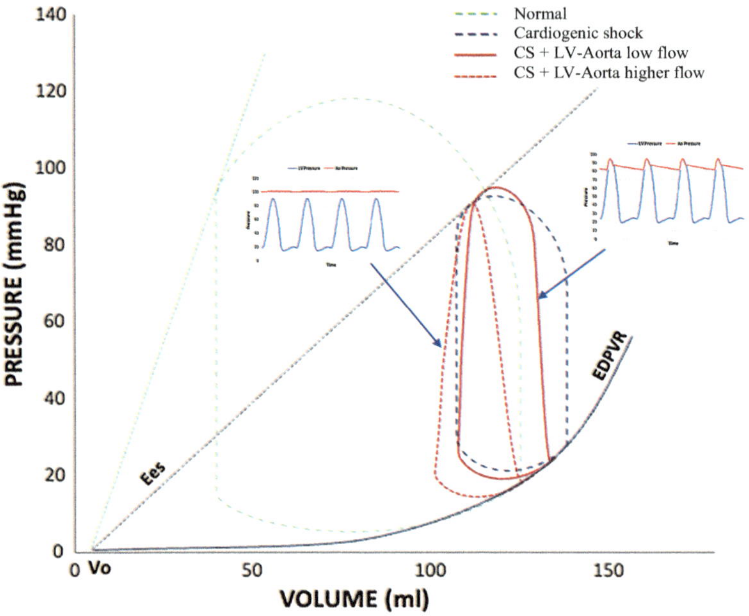

Fig. 11.2 *Cardiogenic shock plus a percutaneous LV to aorta assist device (pLVAD; Impella, Abiomed, Danvers, MA).* These PVLs illustrate the degree of circulatory support and direct unloading of the LV provided by the Impella. The Impella axial flow pump propels blood from either ventricle into the pulmonary artery or aorta in series with the respective ventricle. The device can generate up to ~5 L/min. The continuous pumping of blood directly from the LV, independent of the phase of the cardiac cycle, results in the loss of the normal isovolumic periods and leads to a triangular shaped PVL. In contrast to other MCS devices, removal of blood from the LV is not dependent on ejection through the aortic valve. The Impella markedly improves myocardial energetics. The CPP increases significantly due a rise in aortic diastolic pressure and decrease in LV diastolic pressure. At the same time, the device provides significant LV unloading. The LV PVL is shifted down and to the left indicating a significant decrease in the PVA and myocardial VO_2. The LV EDP is significantly reduced. At a certain flow, LV contractility and loading conditions are such that the LV is unable to generate sufficient pressure to open the aortic valve, resulting in a dissociation between LV and aortic pressure. In contrast to VA ECMO, a VAD-induced increase in CO increases the CVP (not shown), the result of an increase in systemic venous return (see Chap. 5)

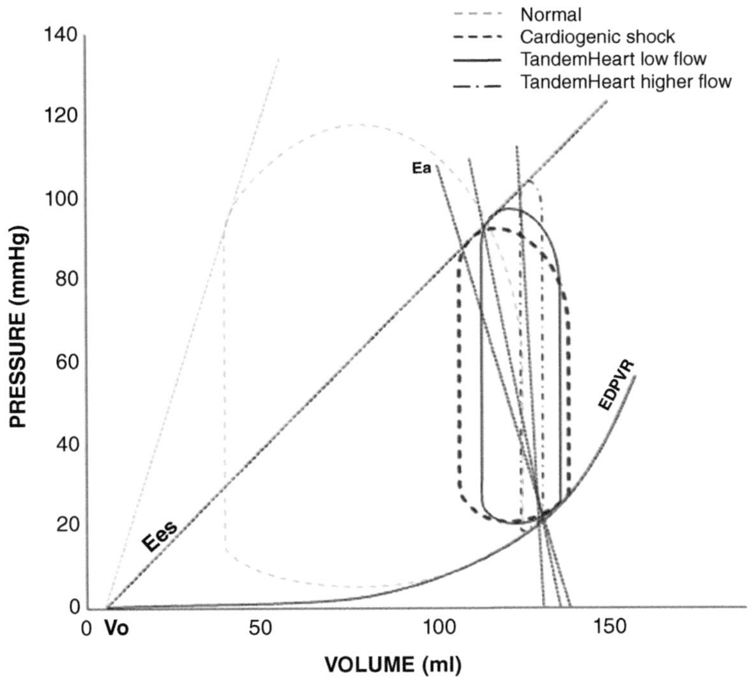

Fig. 11.3 *Cardiogenic shock plus a left atrial to aorta assist device (TandemHeart, Cardiac Assist, Pittsburgh, PA).* These PVLs illustrate the degree of circulatory support and indirect unloading of the LV provided by the TandemHeart. The TandemHeart centrifugal pump and respective ventricle work in parallel, or tandem, by delivering flow to the pulmonary artery or aorta. A membrane oxygenator may be added to the circuit. The device can generate ~5 L/minute of flow. The aortic pressure is increased, the EDV and EDP are reduced, and the CPP increased. However, as with VA ECMO, blood must exit the LV through the aortic valve. As the arterial pressure increases, LV pressure generation must also increase

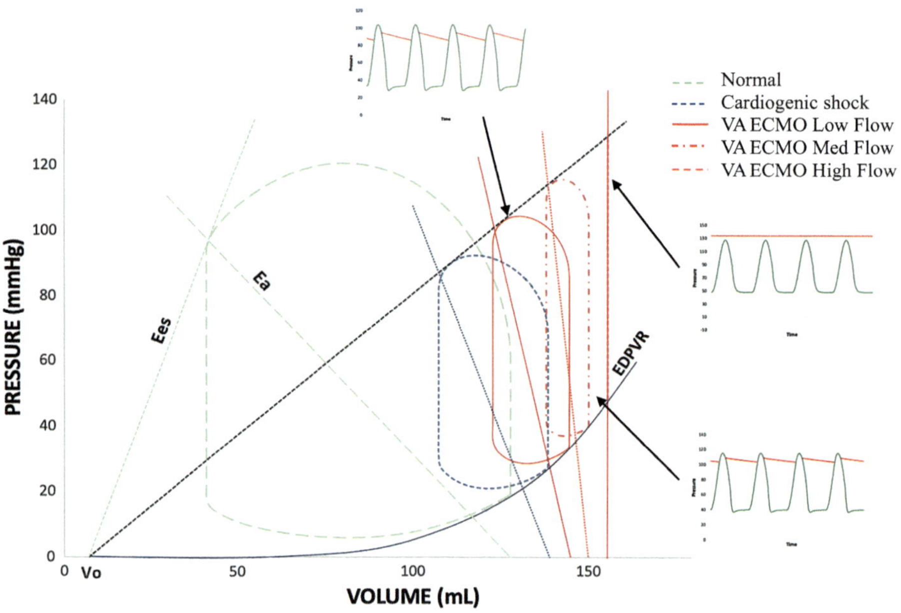

Fig. 11.4 *Cardiogenic shock plus VA ECMO.* VA ECMO provides significant hemodynamic support; however, it does not unload the LV. If VA ECMO flow increases aortic pressure, ventricular afterload and the effective Ea increase. The increase in effective Ea and Ea/Ees, causes the LV EF and SV to decrease and as a result the EDV and EDP to increase. At the same time, persistent RV output, Thesbian drainage, and the return of bronchial blood flow continue to load the LV, with the only egress of blood occurring with ejection through the aortic valve. A new equilibrium is established where LV outflow equals the flow of blood returning to the LV from all sources, and where the increase in arterial pressure necessitates an increase LV pressure generation. As flow is increased further, aortic pressure increases. At a certain flow and afterload, and for a given EDV and inotropic state, the LV is unable to generate adequate pressure to open the aortic valve (the PVL or the far right, which has the appearance of a vertical line), resulting in blood stasis and the dissociation between LV systolic and aortic pressure. With a persistently elevated EDV, the LV remains capable of generating significant pressure albeit less than aortic. Even though there is no LV ejection, the EDV, systolic pressure, and PVA remain significant, as do myocardial VO_2 and the mechanical stress on the LV. The LV EDP remains elevated, leading to ongoing pulmonary edema

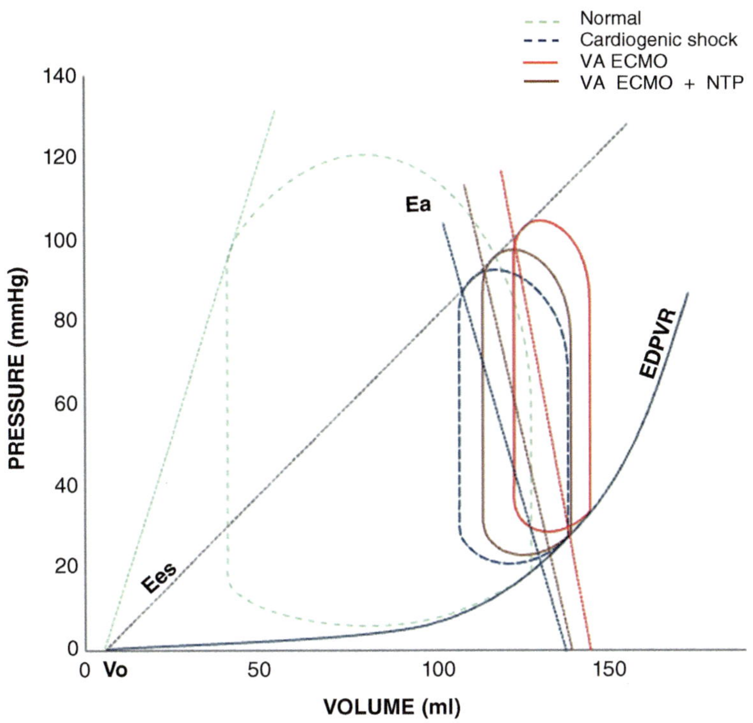

Fig. 11.5 *Cardiogenic shock plus VA ECMO plus vasodilator.* These PVLs illustrate the changes induced by the arterial venous vasodilator NTP. The reduction in Ea and Ea/Ees by NTP causes the EF and SV to increase and the ESV to decrease. The decrease in ESV coupled with NTP-induced venodilation causes the EDV and EDP to decrease. The PVL has been shifted down and to the left, reflecting a significant reduction in LV loading conditions, PVA and myocardial VO_2. And while the aortic diastolic pressure is reduced, an adequate CPP is maintained because of the concomitant significant decrease in EDP

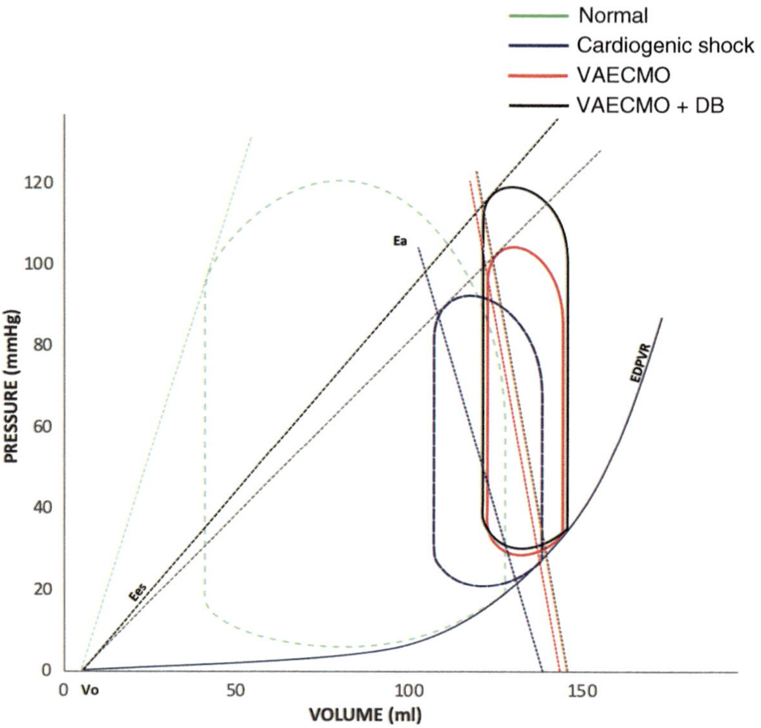

Fig. 11.6 *Cardiogenic shock plus VA ECMO plus an inodilator.* These PVLs illustrate the impact of the inodilator DB. DB decreases SVR however due to the increase in HR, Ea remains unchanged, while Ees has increased. As a result, Ea/Ees decreases, the EF and SV increase. Despite its vasodilatory effect, the increase in Ees without a change in Ea increases the Pes and systolic BP (LV afterload). Myocardial VO_2 increases some 20%, the result of an increase in PVA, calcium cycling (PVA-independent mechanism) and HR. The LV EDP remains significantly elevated

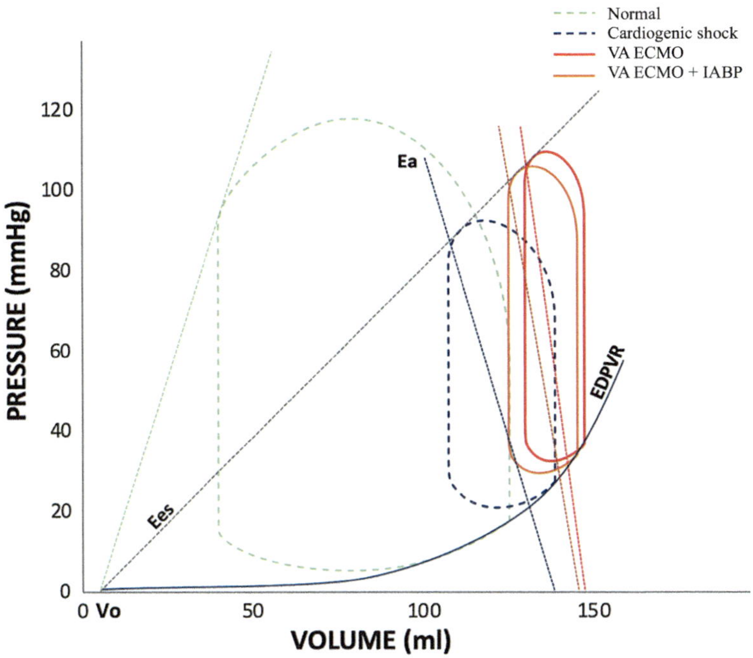

Fig. 11.7 *Cardiogenic shock plus VA ECMO plus IABP.* These PVLs illustrate the hemodynamic impact of the IABP used as a LV decompressive strategy. The extent to which the IABP unloads the LV is limited and is reflected in a minimal shift of the PVL down and to the left. As a result, the PVA and myocardial VO_2 are minimally affected. The LV EDP remains significantly elevated

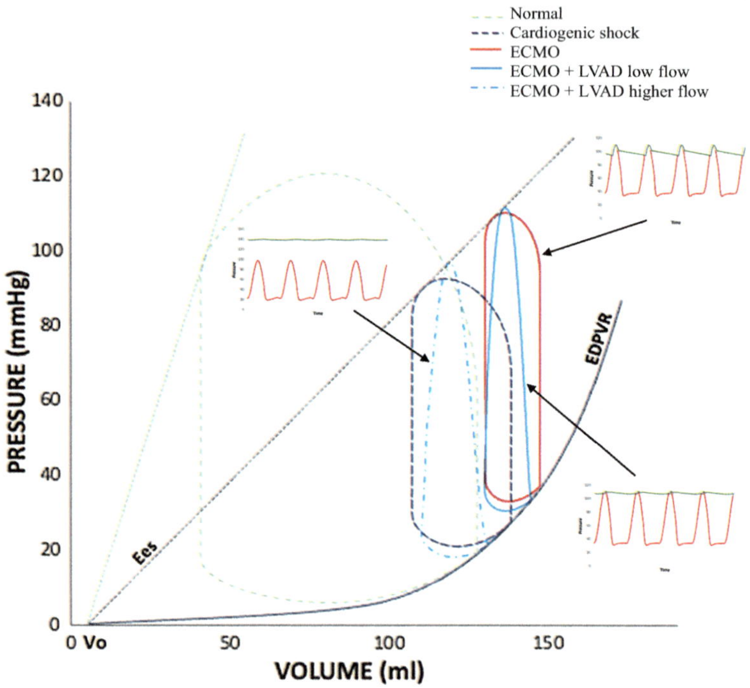

Fig. 11.8 *Cardiogenic shock and VA ECMO plus LVAD. T*hese PVLs illustrate the hemodynamic impact of VA ECMO plus progressive increases in LVAD flow using the percutaneous Impella LVAD (Abiomed, Danvers, MA). The Impella directly unloads the LV, leading to a marked reduction in LV EDV and EDP such that the pressure generating ability of the LV is significantly reduced. This results in the dissociation between LV systolic pressure and aortic pressure. The PVA and myocardial VO_2 are significantly reduced while the CPP increases significantly due to the rise in aortic pressure and decrease in LV diastolic pressure. The myocardial oxygen consumption/delivery relationship is optimized, the mechanical stress on the LV is reduced and the pulmonary capillary hydrostatic pressure is minimized

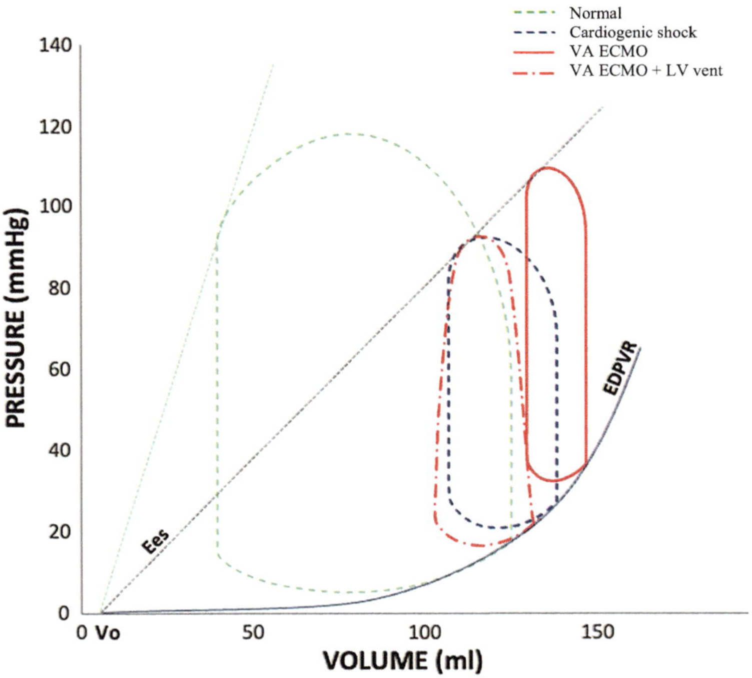

Fig. 11.9 *Cardiogenic shock plus VA ECMO plus LV vent.* These PVLs illustrate the hemodynamic impact of direct unloading of the LV using a vent connected to the inflow cannula of the circuit with flow regulated by a clamp. In this case, the vent is completely unclamped. The LV PVL is shifted appreciably down and to the left, decreasing the PVA and myocardial VO_2. The LV EDP is significantly reduced

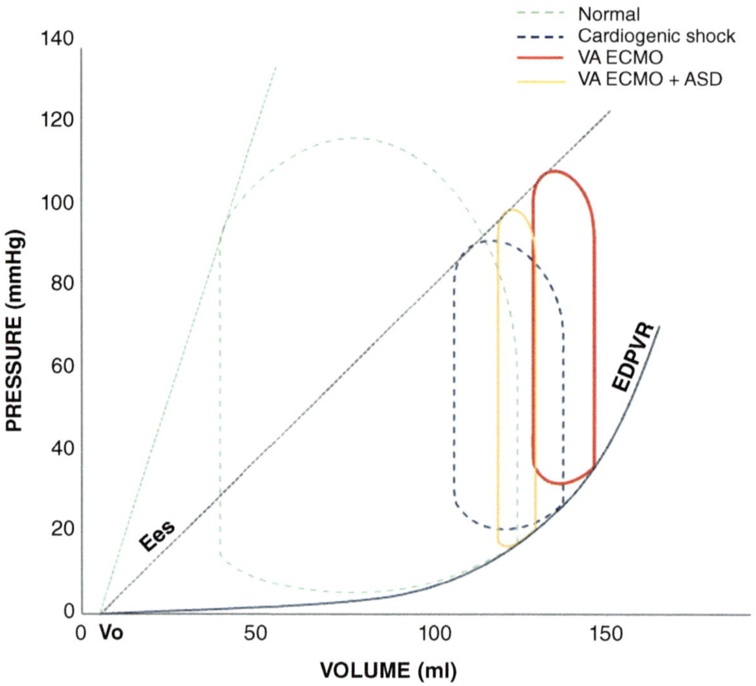

Fig. 11.10 *Cardiogenic shock plus VA ECMO plus an atrial septal defect (ASD).* These PVLs illustrate the hemodynamic impact of a balloon atrial septostomy and the creation of a 10 mm ASD. Percutaneous placement of a left atrial vent connected to the inflow cannula of the circuit is another strategy. Each approach provides effective indirect unloading of the LV, which is reflected in the shift of the PVL down and to the left. The LV EDP is significantly reduced

References

1. Rihal CS, Naidu SS, Givertz MM, et al. 2015 SCAI/ACC/HFSA/STS clinical expert consensus statement on the use of percutaneous mechanical circulatory support devices in cardiovascular care. J Am Coll Cardiol. 2015;65:e7–e26.
2. Telukuntla KS, Estep JD. Acute mechanical circulatory support for cardiogenic shock. Methodist Debakey Cardiovasc J. 2020;16:27–35.
3. Burkhoff D, Sayer G, Doshi D, et al. Hemodynamics of mechanical circulatory support. J Am Coll Cardiol. 2015;23:2663–74.
4. Furer A, Wessler J, Burkhoff D. Hemodynamics of cardiogenic shock. Interv Cardiol Clin. 2017;6:359–71.
5. Rao P, Khalpey Z, Smith R, et al. Venoarterial extracorporeal membrane oxygenation for cardiogenic shock and cardiac arrest. Circ Heart Fail. 2018;11(9):e004905.
6. West JB. Role of the fragility of the pulmonary blood-gas barrier in the evolution of the pulmonary circulation. Am J Physiol Regul Integr Comp Physiol. 2013;304:R171–6.
7. Nugent K, Dobbe L, Rahman R, et al. Lung morphology and surfactant function in cardiogenic pulmonary edema: a narrative review. J Thorac Dis. 2019;11:4031–8.
8. Bachofen H, Schurch S, Michel RP, et al. Experimental hydrostatic pulmonary edema in rabbit lungs. Morphology. Am Rev Respir Dis. 1993;147:989–96.

9. Bachofen H, Schurch S, Weibel ER. Experimental hydrostatic pulmonary edema in rabbit lungs. Barrier lesions. Am Rev Respir Dis. 1993;147:997–1004.
10. Burkhoff D, Naidu SS. The science behind percutaneous hemodynamic support: a review and comparison of support strategies. Catheter Cardiovasc Interv. 2012;80:816–29.
11. Uriel N, Sayer G, Annamalai S, et al. Mechanical unloading in heart failure. J Am Coll Cardiol. 2018;72:569–80.
12. Uchida K, Scarborough EA, Prosser BL. Cardiomyocyte microtubules: control of mechanics, transport, and remodeling. Annu Rev Physiol. 2022;84:257–83.
13. Zhang J, Narula J. Molecular biology of myocardial recovery. Surg Clin N Am. 2004;84:223–42.
14. Meani P, Gelsomino S, Natour E, et al. Modalities and effects of left ventricle unloading on extracorporeal life support: a review of the current literature. Eur J Heart Fail. 2017;19(Suppl 2):84–91.
15. Lorusso R. Are two crutches better than one? The ongoing dilemma on the effects and need for left ventricular unloading during veno-arterial extracorporeal membrane oxygenation. Eur J Heart Fail. 2017;19:413–5.
16. Stewart GC. Finding the right time and place to vent. J Am Coll Cardiol. 2018;6:1044–66.
17. Russo JJ, Aleksova N, Pitcher I, et al. Left ventricular unloading during extracorporeal membrane oxygenation in patients with cardiogenic shock. J Am Coll Cardiol. 2019;73:654–62.
18. Pappalardo F, Schulte C, Pieri M, et al. Concomitant implantation of Impella on top of veno-arterial extracorporeal membrane oxygenation may improve survival of patients with cariogenic shock. Eur J Heart Fail. 2017;19:404–12.
19. Schrage B, Burkhoff D, Rubsamen N, et al. Unloading of the left ventricle during venoarterial extracorporeal membrane oxygenation therapy in cardiogenic shock. JACC Heart Fail. 2018;6:1035–43.
20. Donker DW, Burkhoff D, Mack MJ. ECMO: we need to vent about the need to vent! J Am Coll Cardiol. 2022;79:1251–3.
21. Grandin EW, Nunez JI, Willar B, et al. Mechanical left ventricular unloading in patients undergoing venoarterial extracorporeal membrane oxygenation. J Am Coll Cardiol. 2022;79:1239–50.

Chapter 12
Primary Mitral Regurgitation

Alex Alali and Ronald A. Bronicki

Moderate to severe mitral regurgitation (MR) may present with dyspnea, hemodynamic instability, and shock. An accurate and timely diagnosis can be difficult as the clinical presentation may be nonspecific. Symptoms at presentation may also reflect the underlying pathogenesis of the regurgitant lesion such as endocarditis and sepsis. The presentation depends not only on the severity of the regurgitation but also on whether the regurgitant lesion is acute or chronic, with the latter allowing time for ventricular remodeling and adaptation. For optimal outcomes, a prompt diagnosis with optimal medical therapy is needed. Mechanical circulatory support, percutaneous intervention, or surgery may be indicated, particularly if the lesion is acute and the degree of regurgitation is at least moderate. In this discussion, we review the pathophysiology and impact of vasoactive therapy in the management of acute and chronic MR.

It is important to differentiate the pathophysiological effects of MR due to a primary abnormality of the mitral valve leaflets or their supporting apparatus (primary MR) from those in which the MR is secondary to abnormalities of left ventricular geometry and function (secondary or functional MR). Secondary MR is discussed in the chapter on chronic left ventricular systolic heart failure.

Primary MR may be congenital in origin or result from myocardial ischemia-induced papillary muscle dysfunction, endocarditis, or following a procedure such as balloon valvuloplasty. The presentation of primary MR varies considerably depending on its severity and duration and thus the extent of ventricular remodeling.

A. Alali
University of Pennsylvania Perelman School of Medicine, Children's Hospital of Philadelphia, Philadelphia, PA, USA
e-mail: alalia@chop.edu

R. A. Bronicki (✉)
Baylor College of Medicine, Texas Children's Hospital, Houston, TX, USA
e-mail: rxbronic@texaschildrens.org

R. A. Bronicki et al. (eds.), *Simulation in Cardiovascular Critical Care Medicine*, https://doi.org/10.1007/978-3-031-63557-1_12

In acute severe MR, the rapid development of MR precludes ventricular remodeling, and the regurgitant fraction is greater than 50%. This leads to a significant increase in end diastolic volume and pressure, cardiogenic pulmonary edema, impaired oxygenation and respiratory distress, and a low forward stroke volume and cardiac output and cardiogenic shock. Echocardiography subjectively quantitates the magnitude of the regurgitation, and LV size is minimally elevated. Mild to moderate acute MR may be managed medically, whereas acute, severe MR may be stabilized or temporized by medical therapy but most likely requires surgical intervention.

In chronic compensated MR, the volume load has stimulated structural remodeling of the left ventricle [1–7]. The increase in ventricular diastolic volume, pressure, and wall stress stimulates ventricular remodeling characterized by eccentric hypertrophy. The addition of new sarcomeres in series leads to chamber enlargement and a decrease in diastolic pressure. The increase in left ventricular volume increases systolic wall stress, stimulating concentric hypertrophy. The addition of myofibrils in parallel increases ventricular wall thickness, normalizing the left ventricular wall thickness-to-volume ratio and wall stress.

The marked increase in left ventricular capacitance allows for a significant increase in end diastolic volume and total stroke volume, such that the forward stroke volume and cardiac output approach normal [8–13]. The left atrial pressure remains elevated albeit significantly less than in the acute uncompensated phase due a significant increase in left atrial and ventricular compliance [8–13]. The ejection fraction is greater than normal, as total left ventricular stroke volume (regurgitant and forward stroke volume) increases to a greater extent than the end diastolic volume [13–16].

Decompensation of chronic MR may result from a combination of a decrease in left ventricular contractility or increase in arterial impendence/arterial load or degree of regurgitation. The forward stroke volume and cardiac output decrease, the ejection fraction normalizes or falls below normal, and end systolic and end diastolic volumes and pressure increase from an elevated baseline, leading to pulmonary edema and impaired respiratory function.

Following the repair of chronic MR, there may be an acute increase in ventricular stiffness, as the increased myocardial mass is distributed over a smaller surface area, such that the left ventricular wall thickness-to-volume ratio increases [17–20]. Over the following weeks to months, regression of ventricular hypertrophy leads to a normalization of ventricular geometry and function.

The pressure volume loops shown here (Figs. 12.1, 12.2, 12.3, 12.4, 12.5, and 12.6) illustrate the development of acute MR and the impact of an inoconstrictor and inodilator and chronic MR and ventricular adaptation. The recommendations

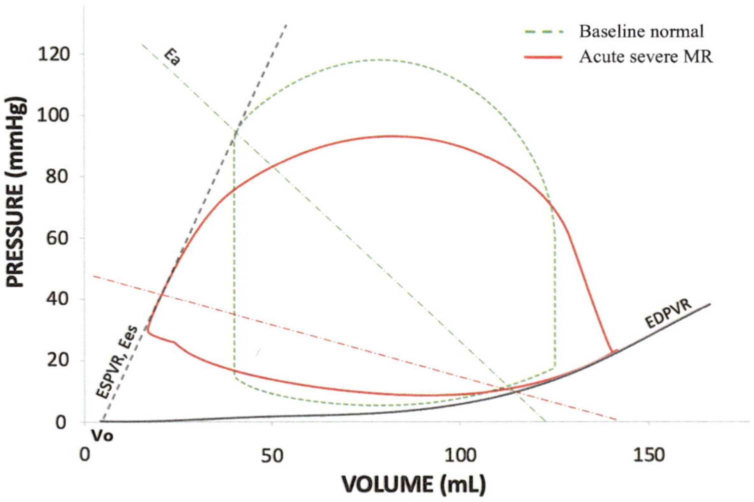

Fig. 12.1 *Acute, severe primary MR.* With MR, the isovolumic contraction phase of the cardiac cycle is absent. LV ejection starts with the regurgitant flow as soon as ventricular pressure rises above left atrial pressure. The isovolumic relaxation phase of the cardiac cycle is absent as well. Following aortic valve closure, regurgitation continues as ventricular pressure is greater than left atrial pressure. Regurgitation reduces LV volume until LV pressure falls below left atrial pressure
In this instance, the MR is severe with a RF (regurgitant volume/total SV) of >50%. The forward SV has decreased by ~50%, resulting in a low CO and BP. The regurgitant volume has increased the EDV and EDP significantly, causing pulmonary edema. In MR, the PAOP (a surrogate measure of mean left atrial pressure) increases to a much greater extent than the EDP (13–26 versus 18–23 mmHg, respectively). Because the MR is acute and severe, the likelihood of effectively temporizing the situation with pharmacologic therapies alone is low
In MR, the forward SV (not apparent in the PVL) or total SV (regurgitant plus forward volumes) may be used to determine Ea [14–16]. Ea based on the total SV ("Ea total") reflects the total afterload on the LV, both the arterial load and low impedance pathway provided by the left atrium (depicted above). Ea based on the forward SV ("Ea forward") determines solely the arterial load. Ea total is considerably lower than Ea for a normal circulation. And because the EF is based on total ventricular afterload (Ea total/Ees), the EF in MR is significantly elevated

from consensus-driven statements on the care of children and adults with cardiogenic shock vary considerably [21–23]. Recommendations for frontline vasoactive agents include inodilators, inoconstrictors, and vasopressors. For these reasons, we have contrasted the hemodynamic impact of these agents. The emphasis is on the *effects* of each agent on the circulation and in turn pressure and flow rather than the *agent or class of agent* selected. The changes in magnitude of the hemodynamic parameters may vary depending on the host response to the therapy.

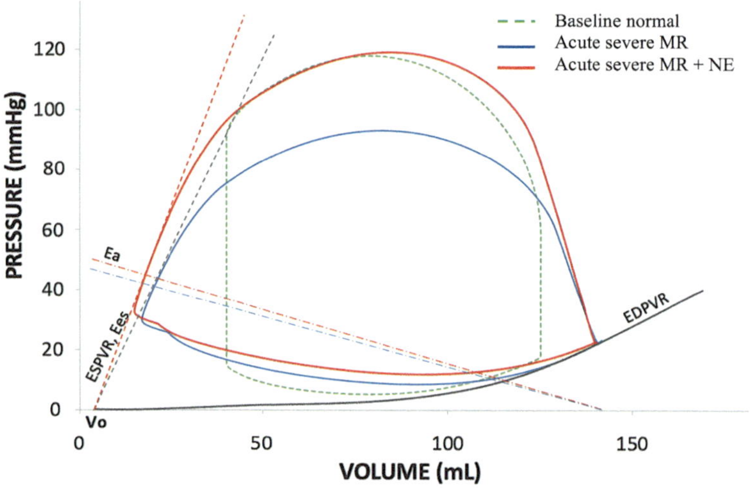

Fig. 12.2 *Inoconstrictor in acute, severe primary mitral MR.* These PVLs illustrate the effects of the inoconstrictor NE in the patient with acute, severe primary MR (RF 66%) discussed in Fig. 12.1. In severe MR, Ea total is very low. Thus, while NE has increased SVR, HR, and Ea forward, Ea total remains very low. Ees increases from a normal baseline. As a result, Ea total/Ees remains very low, the EF very high, and the total SV unchanged. However, because of the increase in Ea forward, the forward SV and CO have decreased further (~15–20%) and the regurgitant volume and RF have increased

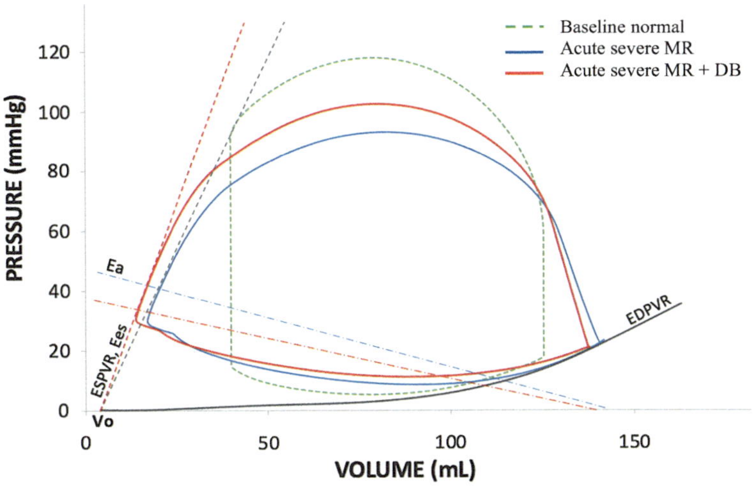

Fig. 12.3 *Inodilator in acute, severe primary MR.* These PVLs illustrate the effects of the inodilator DB in the same patient with acute, severe primary MR. In this instance, DB was titrated to increase contractility to a similar extent as occurred with NE. SVR has decreased to a greater extent than the HR has increased and thus Ea forward has decreased. Ea total remains very low, while Ees increases from a normal baseline. As a result, Ea total/Ees remains very low and total SV unchanged. The decrease in Ea forward causes the forward SV and CO to increase (~10–15%) and the regurgitant volume and RF to decrease

When comparing the inoconstrictor and inodilator strategies, the forward SV and CO are considerably greater (~25%), the regurgitant volume and RF lower with the inodilator. With similar increases in HR, myocardial VO_2 is less with the inodilator due to a smaller PVA (~15%)

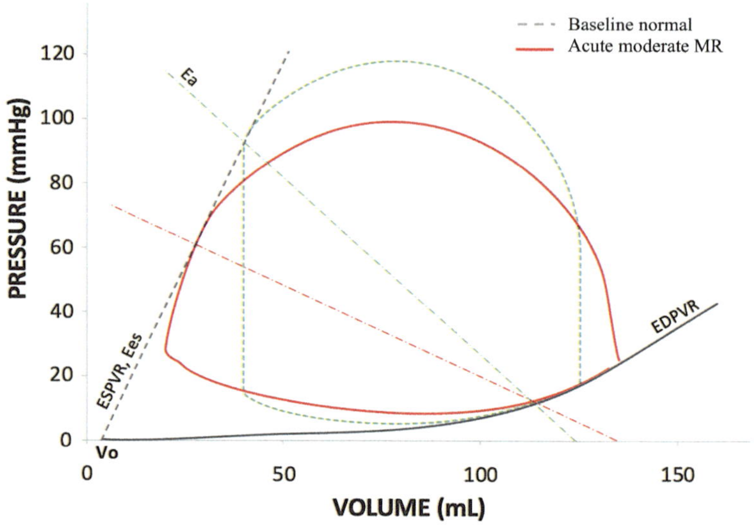

Fig. 12.4 *Acute, moderate primary MR.* These PVLs contrast a normal LV to one with acute, moderate primary MR (RF < 50%). Because the MR is moderate in severity, there is a greater likelihood of effectively temporizing the situation with pharmacologic therapies alone. The decrease in forward SV and CO is far less, and the resulting BP is much greater than in the acute, severe primary MR simulation

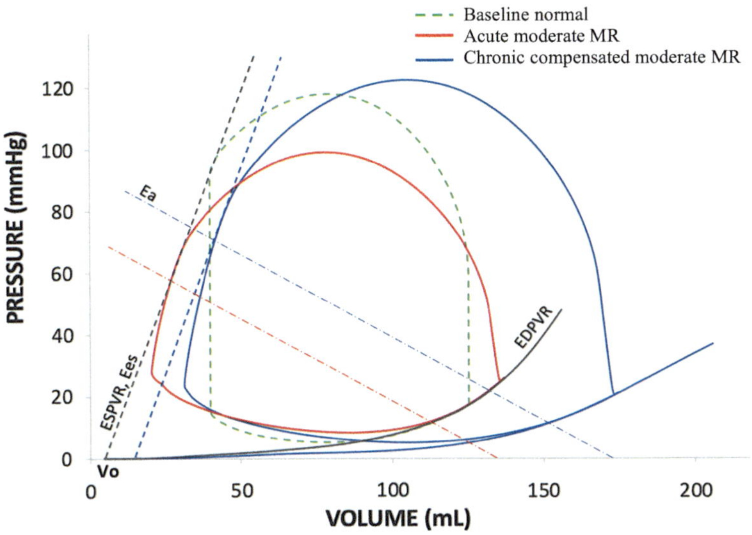

Fig. 12.5 *Chronic, compensated moderate primary MR.* These PVLs illustrate a normal LV, a LV with acute, moderate MR, and a LV with moderate MR that has undergone ventricular remodeling. Comparing chronic compensated to acute uncompensated moderate MR, ventricular stiffness has decreased and Vo and ventricular capacitance have increased (see Chap. 2). Despite a significant increase in the EDV, the EDP is significantly less than in the acute uncompensated state. The significant increase in EDV increases the total SV. As a result, the forward SV and CO have nearly normalized. In this instance, LV contractility has decreased. Although Ees is unchanged, Vo has increased indicating a decrease in end-systolic pressure generation at a common volume. Ea total (depicted) remains very low and thus the EF very high

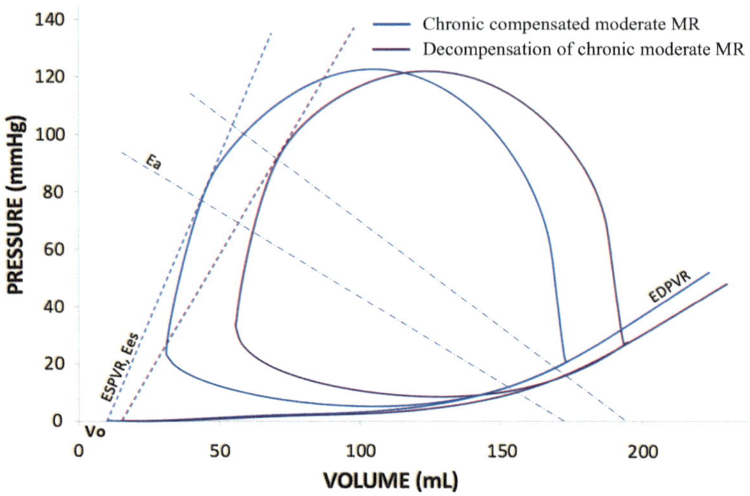

Fig. 12.6 *Decompensation of chronic, moderate primary MR.* These PVLs illustrate a LV with primary MR that has undergone compensatory remodeling followed by decompensation resulting from a decrease in contractility, and neurohormonal activation and an increase in SVR and SBV (see Chap. 5). The severity of the MR has not changed. Ea forward and thus Ea total have increased, Ees has decreased. As a result of the increase in Ea total/Ees, the EF and total SV have decreased. The increase in Ea forward maintains the BP despite the decrease in forward SV. The EF remains greater than normal (73%) despite the appreciable decrease in contractility because Ea total and Ea total/Ees remain low. Despite a further decrease in ventricular stiffness, the EDP has increased due to the large increase in SBV and in turn LV EDV

References

1. Glantz SA, Parmley WW. Factors which affect the diastolic pressure-volume curve. Circ Res. 1978;42:171–80.
2. Mirsky I, Pasipoularides A. Clinical assessment of diastolic function. Prog Cardiovasc Dis. 1990;4:291–318.
3. Gaasch WH. Left ventricular radius to wall thickness ratio. Am J Cardiol. 1979;43:1189–94.
4. Gaasch WH, Levine HJ, Quinones MA, et al. Left ventricular compliance: mechanisms and clinical implications. Am J Cardiol. 1976;38:645–53.
5. Gaasch WH, Zile MR. Ventricular structural remodeling in health and disease. J Am Coll Cardiol. 2011;58:1733–40.
6. Grossman W, Paulus WJ. Myocardial stress and hypertrophy: a complex interface between biophysics and cardiac remodeling. J Clin Invest. 2013;123(9):3701–3.
7. Grossman W. Cardiac hypertrophy: useful adaptation or pathologic process. Am J Med. 1980;69:576–84.
8. Carabello BA, Crawford FA Jr. Valvular heart disease. N Engl J Med. 1997;337:32–41.
9. Gaasch WH, Meyer TE. Left ventricular response to mitral regurgitation: implications for management. Circulation. 2008;118:2298–303.
10. Stout KK, Verrier ED. Acute valvular regurgitation. Circulation. 2009;119:3232–41.
11. Carabello BA. The current therapy for mitral regurgitation. J Am Coll Cardiol. 2008;52:319–26.
12. Bastos MB, Burkhoff D, Maly J, et al. Invasive left ventricle pressure-volume analysis: overview and practical clinical implications. Eur Heart J. 2020;41:1286–97.

13. Burkhoff D. Pressure-volume loops in clinical research. J Am Coll Cardiol. 2013;62:1173–6.
14. Osuga T, Morita T, Sasaki N, et al. Prognostic value of left ventricular-arterial coupling estimated using echocardiography in dogs with myxomatous mitral valve disease. J Vet Intern Med. 2021;35:2607–15.
15. Starling MR. Left ventricular pump efficiency in long-term mitral regurgitation assessed by means of left ventricular-arterial coupling relations. Am Heart J. 1994;127:1324–35.
16. Imasaka K, Tayama E, Tomita Y. Left ventricular performance early after repair for posterior mitral leaflet prolapse: chordal replacement versus leaflet resection. J Thorac Cardiovasc Surg. 2015;150:538–45.
17. Zile MR, Tomita M, Ishihara K, et al. Changes in diastolic function during development and correction of chronic LV volume overload produced by mitral regurgitation. Circulation. 1993;87:1378–88.
18. Zaid R, Barker CM, Little SH, et al. Pre- and post-operative diastolic dysfunction in patients with valvular heart disease. J Am Coll Cardiol. 2013;62:1922–30.
19. Lavall D, Reil J-C, Schmitz L, et al. Early hemodynamic improvement after percutaneous mitral valve repair evaluated by noninvasive pressure-volume analysis. J Am Soc Echocardiogr. 2016;29:888–98.
20. Gaemperli O, Biaggi P, Gugelmann R, et al. Real-time left ventricular pressure-volume loops during percutaneous mitral valve repair with the MitraClip system. Circulation. 2013;127:1018–27.
21. Law YM, Lal AK, Chen S, et al. Diagnosis and management of myocarditis in children. A scientific statement from the American heart association. Circulation. 2021;144:e123–35.
22. Van Diepen S, Katz JN, Albert NM, et al. Contemporary management of cardiogenic shock. A scientific statement from the American heart association. Circulation. 2017;136:e232–68.
23. Heidenreich PA, Bozkurt B, Aguilar D, et al. 2022 AHA/ACC/HFSA guideline for the management of heart failure: a report of the American college of cardiology/American heart association joint committee on clinical practice guidelines. Circulation. 2022;145:e895–e1032.

Chapter 13
Aortic Regurgitation

Khayri Shalhoub and Ronald A. Bronicki

Moderate to severe acute regurgitation (AR) may present with dyspnea, hemodynamic instability, and shock. An accurate and timely diagnosis can be difficult as the clinical presentation may be nonspecific. Symptoms at presentation may also reflect the underlying pathogenesis of the regurgitant lesion such as endocarditis and sepsis. The presentation depends not only on the severity of the regurgitation but also on whether the regurgitant lesion is acute or chronic, with the latter allowing time for ventricular remodeling and adaptation. For optimal outcomes, a prompt diagnosis with optimal medical therapy is needed. Mechanical circulatory support, percutaneous intervention, or surgery may be indicated, particularly if the lesion is acute and the degree of regurgitation is at least moderate [1]. This is particularly true for AR, where an elevated left ventricular (LV) diastolic pressure is accompanied by decreased aortic diastolic pressure. The decrease in coronary perfusion pressure is compounded by a significant increase in LV myocardial oxygen consumption. In this discussion, we review the pathophysiology and impact of vasoactive therapy in the management of acute and chronic AR.

AR results from diseases of the aortic leaflets or the aortic root (annulus, sinuses, sinotubular junction, and proximal ascending aorta) that distort the leaflets and prevents their coaptation. Aortic root disease occurs in Marfan, Ehlers-Danlos, and Turner syndromes. Common causes of leaflet abnormalities are endocarditis and procedural-related complications (e.g., following balloon valvuloplasty). AR may be associated with congenital heart disease, including bicuspid aortic valves.

K. Shalhoub · R. A. Bronicki (✉)
Baylor College of Medicine, Texas Children's Hospital, Houston, TX, USA
e-mail: kxshalho@texaschildrens.org; rxbronic@texaschildrens.org

R. A. Bronicki et al. (eds.), *Simulation in Cardiovascular Critical Care Medicine*, https://doi.org/10.1007/978-3-031-63557-1_13

Acute AR differs from chronic AR for several reasons. In acute AR, the ventricle has not had time to remodel, and the regurgitant volume leads to a marked increase in LV diastolic pressure and pulmonary edema [2–7]. Severely elevated LV diastolic pressure may also cause premature closure of the mitral valve and diastolic mitral regurgitation. The forward stroke volume, cardiac output, and systolic blood pressure are low. However, the pulse pressure may be wide due to regurgitation into the LV during diastole [8].

This contrasts with chronic AR, where the volume load leads to eccentric hypertrophy and a marked increase in LV capacity and decrease in ventricular stiffness [9]. This significantly increases the total stroke volume, and despite a large regurgitant fraction, the LV can generate a normal forward stroke volume and cardiac output. And despite a significant increase in LV end diastolic volume, the end diastolic pressure is greatly reduced compared to acute AR due to ventricular remodeling. The large total stroke volume is entirely ejected into the aorta, increasing aortic pressure and LV afterload inducing compensatory concentric hypertrophy. Systolic hypertension is accompanied by a wide pulse pressure.

Clinical decompensation in the patients with chronic AR may result from a combination of a decrease in LV contractility, increase in arterial load, or the degree of regurgitation. Decompensation may be associated with an increase in ventricular stiffness [9, 10]. The forward stroke volume and cardiac output decrease, the ejection fraction normalizes or falls below normal, and end systolic and end diastolic volumes and pressure increase from an elevated baseline, leading to pulmonary edema and impaired respiratory function.

Immediately following the repair of chronic AR, there may be an increase in ventricular stiffness due to the acute increase in the ventricular muscle mass-to-end diastolic volume ratio [9, 10]. Over the following weeks to months, regression of ventricular hypertrophy may lead to a normalization of ventricular geometry and stiffness [11, 12].

The recommendations from consensus-driven statements on the care of children and adults with cardiogenic shock vary considerably [13–15]. Recommendations for frontline vasoactive agents include inodilators, inoconstrictors, and vasopressors. For these reasons, we have contrasted the impact of these agents. The emphasis is on the *effects* of each agent on the circulation and in turn pressure and flow rather than the *agent or class of agent* selected. The changes in magnitude of the hemodynamic parameters may vary depending on the host response to the therapy. The following pressure volume loops (Figs. 13.1, 13.2, 13.3, 13.4, 13.5, 13.6, and 13.7) illustrate the development of acute AR of varying severity and the impact of an inoconstrictor and inodilator and ventricular adaptation to chronic AR.

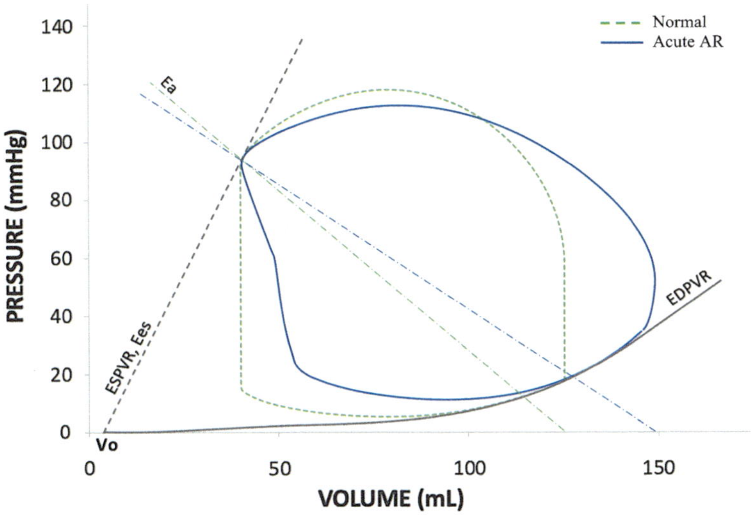

Fig. 13.1 *Acute, moderate to severe AR*. These PVLs illustrate the development of acute, moderate to severe AR. With AR, the isovolumic contraction phase of the cardiac cycle is absent. LV volume continues to increase because as the LV begins to contract and generate pressure, blood is still entering the LV from the aorta because aortic pressure is higher than LV pressure. Once LV pressure exceeds aortic diastolic pressure, the ventricle begins to eject blood into the aorta. The isovolumic relaxation phase of the cardiac cycle is absent as well because as the LV relaxes, blood flows from the aorta into the ventricle. Once the mitral valve opens, filling occurs from the left atrium; however, blood continues to flow from the aorta into the LV throughout diastole because aortic pressure is higher than ventricular pressure

In this simulation, the AR is moderate to severe with a RF of 57%. The forward SV has decreased by ~45%. The regurgitant volume has increased the EDV and EDP significantly resulting in pulmonary edema. In AR, the EDP increases to a much greater extent than the PAOP (18–35 and 13–21 mmHg, respectively). The CPP is marginal due to the elevated EDP and diastolic hypotension. The increase in pulse pressure is limited in acute AR

With AR, the forward or total SV (regurgitant plus forward) may be used to determine Ea. Ea based on the total SV ("Ea total") reflects the total afterload on the LV. Ea based on the forward SV determines solely the arterial load. And because the EF is based on the total ventricular afterload, the EF in AR is elevated

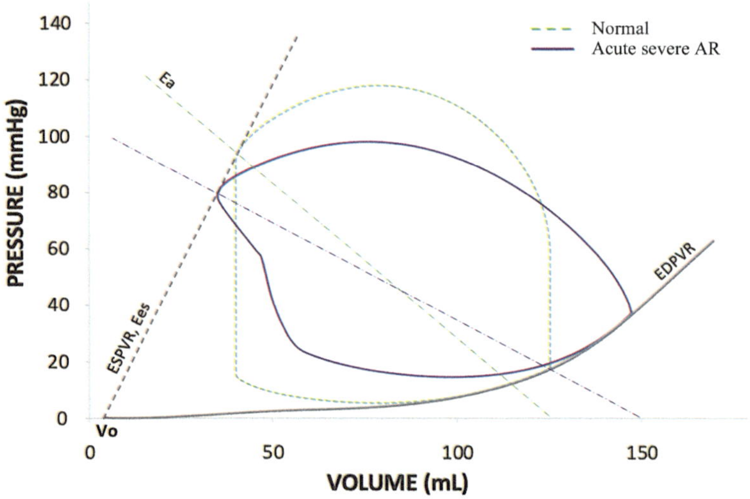

Fig. 13.2 *Acute, severe AR.* These PVLs illustrate the development of acute, severe AR with a regurgitant fraction of 68%. In comparison to the simulation of moderate AR in Fig. 13.1, the forward SV and BP are severely diminished, the EDP further elevated. The CPP is inadequate. In severe AR, the aortic diastolic pressure and ventricular EDP equilibrate, and the elevated EDP results in early mitral valve closure. Because the AR is acute and severe, it is unlikely that pharmacologic therapies alone will effectively temporize the situation

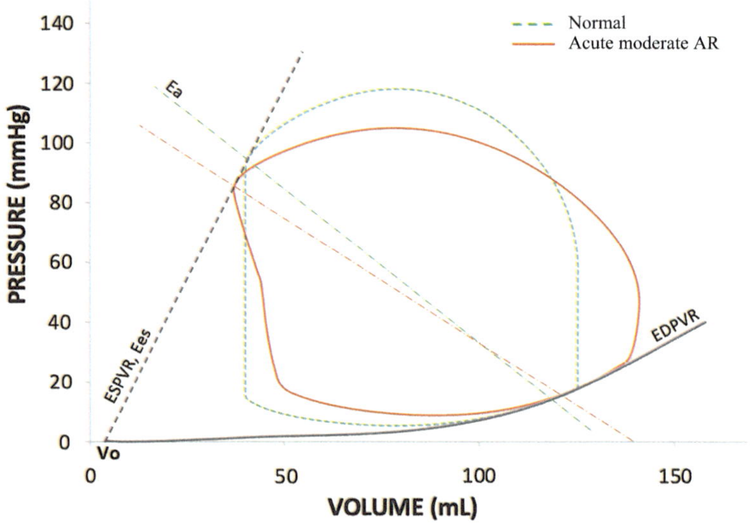

Fig. 13.3 *Acute, moderate AR.* These PVLs illustrate the development of acute, moderate AR (RF 48%). Prior to the initiation of a vasoactive agent, Ea total is reduced (Pes is reduced, total SV elevated). This coupled with a normal Ees causes the Ea total/Ees to be less than normal, the EF to be elevated (74%). Because the AR is moderate in severity, there is a greater likelihood of effectively temporizing the situation with pharmacologic therapies alone

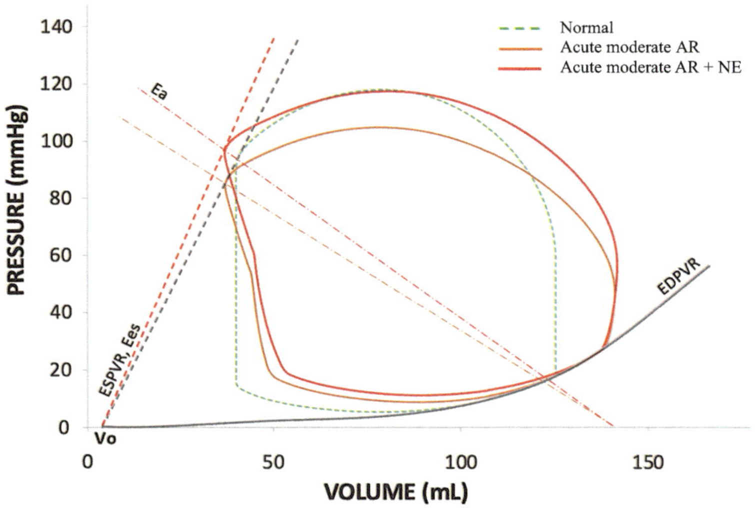

Fig. 13.4 *Acute, moderate AR treated with an inoconstrictor.* These PVL illustrate the impact of the inoconstrictor NE in the patient with acute moderate AR from Fig. 13.3. NE increases the Ea forward and thus total Ea, and Ees. Ea total/Ees is unchanged and thus the total SV is unchanged. The increase in Ea forward decreases the forward SV (~10%), and increases the RF

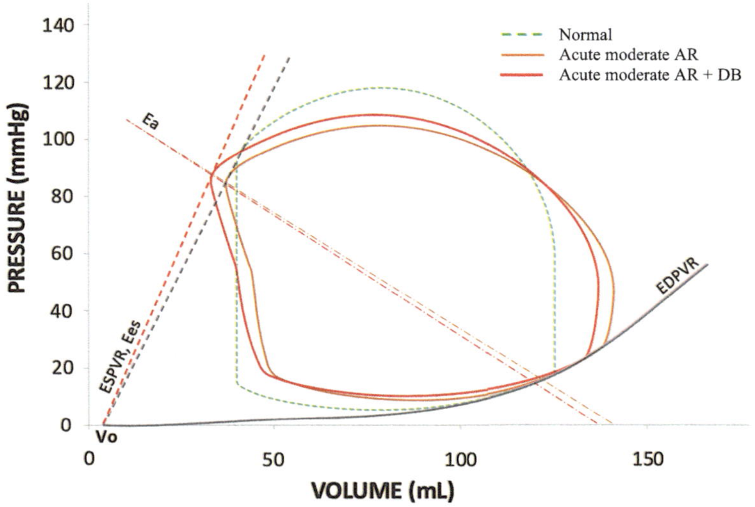

Fig. 13.5 *Acute, moderate AR treated with an inodilator.* These PVLs illustrate the impact of the inodilator DB in the same patient with acute moderate AR discussed in Figs. 13.3 and 13.4. DB decreases SVR but also increases the HR. The net effect is little change in Ea forward. DB has been titrated to increase Ees to the same extent as occurred with NE in Fig. 13.3. Ees increases, and Ea total/Ees decreases. However, the impact of this on the total SV is offset by venodilation and a decrease in SBV and ultimately EDV (as well as EDP). As a result, despite an increase in the EF, the total SV is unchanged

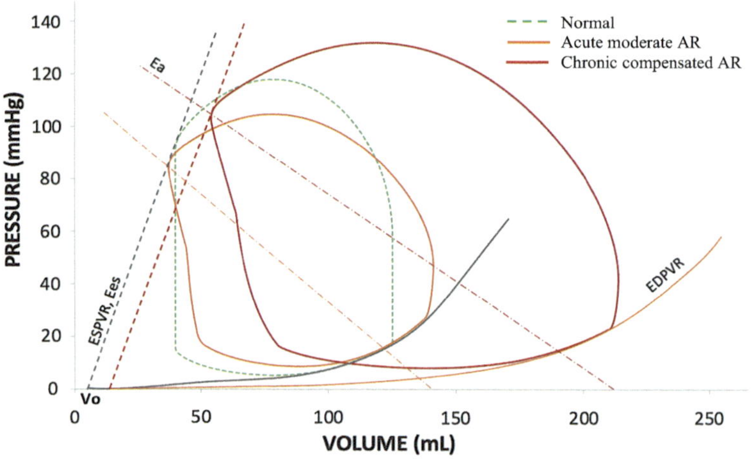

Fig. 13.6 *Chronic compensated AR.* These PVLs illustrate the progression from the development of acute, moderate AR to chronic compensated AR. In response to the volume load, the LV has undergone eccentric hypertrophy, significantly increasing its capacity. As a result, the total SV is significantly elevated, and the forward SV approaches normal. Due to the significant increase in total SV, the BP and pulse pressure have increased significantly. The subsequent increase in systolic pressure and ventricular afterload stimulates concentric hypertrophy as well. The EDV has increased considerably; however, the EDP is only mildly elevated due to a marked decrease in ventricular stiffness. This is reflected in a shift of the EDPVR down and to the right. Ees is elevated; however, overall contractility is diminished due to the increase in Vo, where diminished contractility is indicated by a decrease in systolic pressure generation at a common volume

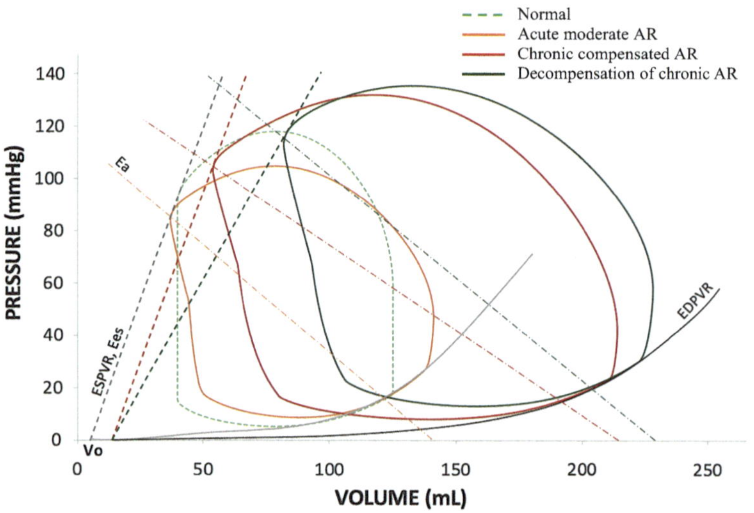

Fig. 13.7 *Decompensation of chronic AR.* These PVLs illustrate the decompensation of chronic AR in the same patient discussed in Fig. 13.6. In this case, decompensation results from a decrease in contractility (Ees has decreased, Vo remains unchanged), increase in Ea forward (SVR and HR), and increase in SBV. The Ea total/Ees has increased, and the EF and total SV have decreased. The EDP has risen considerably due to the increase in ESV and SBV

References

1. Bernard S, Deferm S, Bertrand PB. Acute valvular emergencies. Eur Heart J Acute Cardiovasc Care. 2022;11:653–65.
2. Bastos MB, Burkhoff D, Maly J, et al. Invasive left ventricle pressure-volume analysis: overview and practical clinical implications. Eur Heart J. 2020;41:1286–97.
3. Devlin WH, Petrusha J, Briesmiester BS, et al. Impact of vascular adaptation to chronic aortic regurgitation on left ventricular performance. Circulation. 1999;99:1027–33.
4. Gaasch WH, Sundaram M, Meyer TE. Managing asymptomatic patients with chronic aortic regurgitation. Chest. 1997;111:1702–9.
5. Stout KK, Verrier ED. Acute valvular regurgitation. Circulation. 2009;119:3232–41.
6. Carabello BA, Crawford FA Jr. Valvular heart disease. N Engl J Med. 1997;337:32–41.
7. Voit J, Otto CM, Burke CR. Acute native aortic regurgitation: clinical presentation, diagnosis and management. Heart. 2022;108:1651–60.
8. Mann T, McLaurin L, Grossman W, et al. Assessing the hemodynamic severity of acute aortic regurgitation due to infective endocarditis. N Engl J Med. 1975;293:108–13.
9. Gaasch WH, Zile MR. Left ventricular structural remodeling in health and disease. J Am Coll Cardiol. 2011;58:1733–40.
10. Zaid RR, Barker CM, Little SH, et al. Pre- and post-operative diastolic dysfunction in patients with valvular heart disease. J Am Coll Cardiol. 2013;62:1922–30.
11. Lamb HJ, Beyerbacht HP, de Roos A, et al. Left ventricular remodeling early after aortic valve replacement: differential effects on diastolic function in aortic valve stenosis and aortic regurgitation. J Am Coll Cardiol. 2002;40:2182–8.
12. Villari B, Sossalla S, Quirino C, et al. Persistent diastolic dysfunction late after valve replacement in severe aortic regurgitation. Circulation. 2009;120:2386–92.
13. Maconochie IK, Aickin R, Hazinski MF, et al. Pediatric life support. 2020 international consensus on cardiopulmonary resuscitation and emergency cardiovascular care science with treatment recommendations. Circulation. 2020;142(suppl 1):S140–84.
14. van Diepen S, Katz JN, Albert NM, et al. Contemporary management of cardiogenic shock. A scientific statement from the American Heart Association. Circulation. 2017;136:e232–68.
15. Levy B, Bastien O, Bendjelid K, et al. Experts' recommendations for the management of adult patients with cardiogenic shock. Ann Intensive Care. 2015;5(17):1–10.

Chapter 14
Aortic Valve Stenosis

Jordan Schneider and Ronald A. Bronicki

Aortic valve stenosis may result from hypoplasia of the aortic valve annulus and/or abnormalities of the valve leaflets [1–4]. Congenital aortic valve stenosis may be associated with other cardiovascular abnormalities, including hypoplasia of left heart structures, subvalvar stenosis (fixed or dynamic), and supravalvar obstruction. Calcification of the aortic valve leaflets contributes importantly to the pathophysiology of aortic stenosis [5]. Calcification develops because of mechanical stress-induced endothelial damage and lipid accumulation followed by fibrosis, leaflet thickening, and ultimately calcification. Progressive narrowing of the aortic valve orifice and pressure loading of the left ventricle (LV) leads to ventricular remodeling.

Over time, the pressure load on the LV results in concentric hypertrophy and an increase LV contractility and myocardial oxygen demand. Concentric hypertrophy also increases the ventricular muscles mass-to-end diastolic volume ratio, increasing ventricular stiffness. The compressive effects of the hypertrophied myocardium may adversely affect coronary perfusion pressure and myocardial oxygenation, particularly in the subendocardial region. This leads to interstitial fibrosis and impaired myocardial relaxation, both of which contribute to diastolic dysfunction.

Decompensation and symptoms of heart failure in aortic stenosis may result from diastolic dysfunction, systolic dysfunction and/or an increase in the effective afterload resulting from an increase in valvular obstruction, peripheral arterial

J. Schneider
Central Michigan University College of Medicine, Children's Hospital of Michigan, Detroit, MI, USA
e-mail: jschneid@dmc.org

R. A. Bronicki (✉)
Baylor College of Medicine, Texas Children's Hospital, Houston, TX, USA
e-mail: rxbronic@texaschildrens.org

R. A. Bronicki et al. (eds.), *Simulation in Cardiovascular Critical Care Medicine*, https://doi.org/10.1007/978-3-031-63557-1_14

resistance, or a decrease in peripheral arterial compliance (an associated finding in aortic stenosis). Following aortic valve intervention and relief of the pressure load, ventricular stiffness remains elevated. Over time, the LV remodels and the ventricular muscle mass or thickness-to-EDV ratio decreases. As a result, ventricular stiffness decreases significantly.

The severity of the obstruction may be assessed by determining one or more of several parameters [6–10]. The peak and mean pressure gradients may be derived by Doppler echocardiography and the peak-to-peak gradient directly measured by cardiac catheterization, with catheterization measurements less than Doppler-derived values because of pressure recovery. The aortic valve area may be assessed by planimetry using echocardiography; however, much greater accuracy is provided by computed tomography or magnetic resonance imaging. The aortic valve area may also be derived from the Gorlin formula (utilizing cardiac catheterization data) and continuity equation (utilizing data from two-dimensional and Doppler echocardiography).

Importantly, there may be discordance between the aortic valve area and hemodynamic parameters because blood flow velocities and pressure gradients are flow dependent. When LV systolic function is reduced, and in turn, stroke volume, the velocity and thus pressure gradient are relatively low despite a small valve area. An increase in the arterial load, due to an increase in peripheral arterial resistance and/or decrease in arterial compliance, contributes importantly to the effective arterial load provided by the stenotic valve because resistance in series is additive. This increase in arterial load decreases transvalvar flow particularly if LV contractility is diminished [11, 12]. The pressure gradient may be relatively low despite the presence of a severely reduced aortic valve area and preserved systolic function (ejection fraction). In this setting, flow is limited due to severe compensatory ventricular hypertrophy and low end diastolic volume. The pressure gradient may be disproportionately high relative to the valve areas due to excessive flow, as seen with concomitant aortic regurgitation or shunt lesion. Finally, the calculated valve area may be lower than actual when the LV is unable to generate sufficient energy to overcome the inertia required to open the valve to its maximum possible extent.

The subsequent pressure volume loops (Figs. 14.1, 14.2, 14.3, 14.4, 14.5, 14.6, and 14.7) illustrate the hemodynamic profiles of compensated aortic stenosis and hemodynamic profiles of decompensated aortic stenosis and the impact of vasoactive therapies. The emphasis is on the *effects* of each agent on the circulation and in turn pressure and flow rather than the *agent or class of agent* selected. The changes in magnitude of the hemodynamic parameters may vary depending on the host response to the therapy. As discussed in Chap. 2, the derivation of Ea is based on assumptions including Pes approximates mean arterial pressure. Due to the nature of aortic stenosis, the elastance model has not been validated.

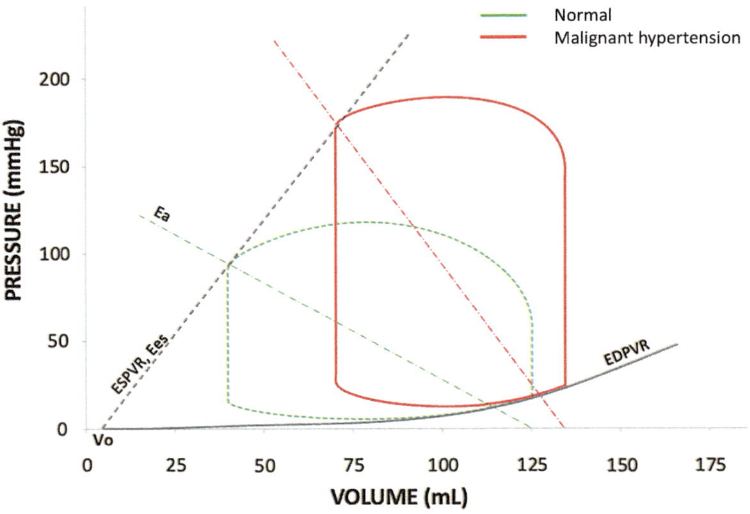

Fig. 14.1 *Acute increase in systemic arterial load.* These PVLs illustrate the effects of an acute increase in arterial load on the LV as seen, for example, in malignant hypertension. Figures 14.2, 14.3, 14.4, 14.5, 14.6, and 14.7 illustrate the impact of chronic increases in the effective arterial load on the LV. In this instance, Ea has increased significantly primarily due to a marked increase in SVR, and to a lesser extent HR. As a result, Ea/Ees is significantly elevated, and the EF falls out of the normal range despite normal contractility. The increase in ESV coupled with neurohormonal activation-induced venoconstriction and increase in SBV, increase the EDV and EDP, resulting in cardiogenic pulmonary edema. The increase in SBV, systemic venous return, and in turn EDV mitigate the decrease in SV resulting from ventricular arterial uncoupling. The marked increased in PVA and to a lesser extent HR have caused myocardial VO_2 to double from baseline

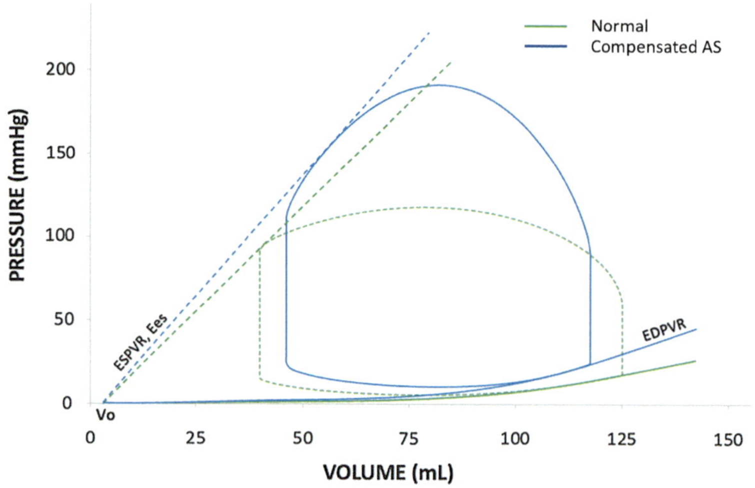

Fig. 14.2 *Chronic compensated AS.* These PVLs illustrate the compensatory response of the LV to a chronically elevated LV afterload due to AS. The aortic valve effective orifice area is 0.8 cm^2 and has resulted in mean and peak transvalvar pressure gradients of 50 and 84 mmHg, respectively. In this case, the increase in LV afterload results from the valvular load (valvar stenosis) as well as arterial load (elevated SVR and decreased arterial compliance). LV afterload (peak LV systolic pressure) in this simulation is similar to the afterload in Fig. 14.1
The chronic increase in LV afterload has induced ventricular remodeling, resulting in concentric hypertrophy and a significant increase in LV Ees. As a result of the commensurate increase in LV contractility, the EF is normal. The SV is less than normal due to a decrease in EDV. Ventricular muscle mass and thickness has increased relative to the EDV, increasing ventricular stiffness. This change is reflected in the shift of the EDPVR up and to left relative to the normal PVL. Despite the decrease in EDV, the EDP exceeds 20 mmHg. Due to the chronicity of the pulmonary venous hypertension and adaptative changes within the pulmonary microvasculature and lymphatics, extravascular lung water formation is limited, and oxygenation is normal. Myocardial VO_2 is some 30–35% greater than for a normal LV due to changes in PVA and PVA-independent factors

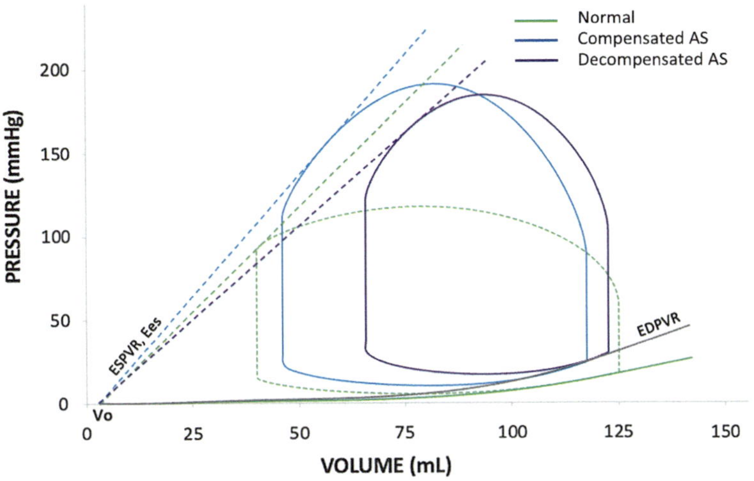

Fig. 14.3 *Decompensation of chronic AS with a maintained BP*. These PVLs illustrate findings consistent with a transition from compensated to decompensated AS due to a decrease in contractility (Ees) from an elevated baseline. The decrement in function has resulted in neurohormonal activation and an increase in SVR and arterial BP as well as TBV and SBV (see Chap. 5). The decrease in LV contractility coupled with an increase in the arterial load causes the EF and SV to decrease, the ESV to increase. Due to the decrease in SV and increase in arterial load, the mean and peak transvalvar pressure gradients have decreased by ~20%. The increase in ESV and SBV increases the EDV and EDP

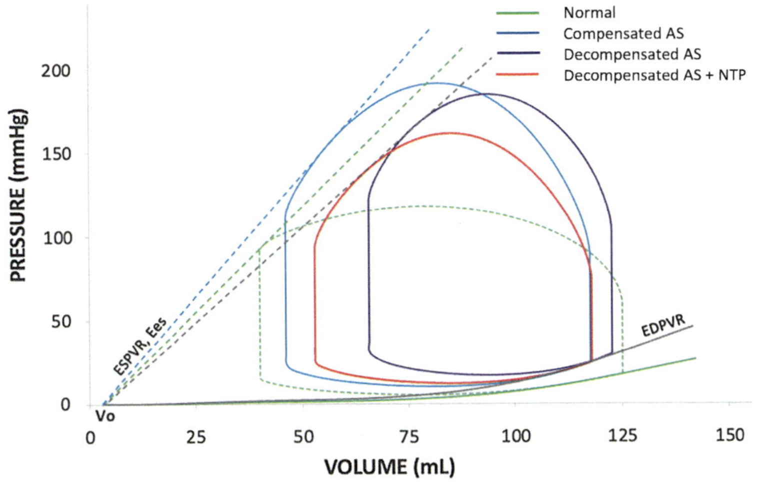

Fig. 14.4 *Decompensated chronic AS with a maintained BP treated with a vasodilator*. These PVLs illustrate the effects of the arterial-venous vasodilator NTP. NTP reduces SVR and the arterial load, decreasing the BP from 123/105 to 95/75 mmHg. As a result, the EF and SV (~15%) increase. In this case, an adequate BP and CPP (>50 mmHg) are maintained. The latter due in part to a decrease in the LV EDP resulting from a decrease in ESV and SBV. Meanwhile, myocardial VO_2 (PVA-related) is reduced

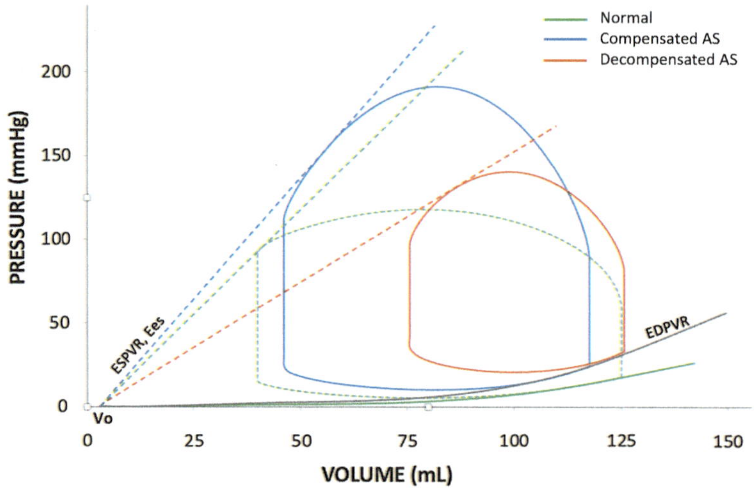

Fig. 14.5 *Decompensation of chronic AS with a marginal BP.* These PVLs illustrate findings consistent with a transition from compensated to decompensated AS due to a much greater decrement in LV contractility than in the previous simulations discussed in Figs. 14.3 and 14.4. Neurohormonal activation has occurred to a similar degree. Ees has decreased to a much greater extent than SVR, and the arterial load has increased, resulting in a marginal BP (98/82 mmHg). The CPP is marginal, and the EDP has risen considerately from an elevated baseline to 32 mmHg

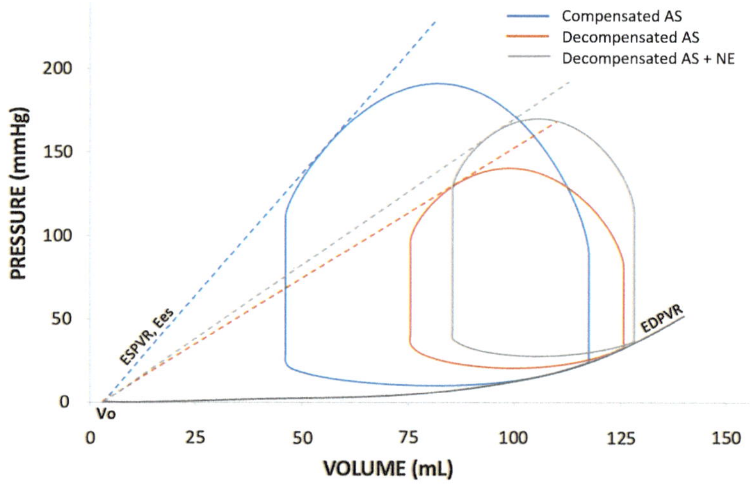

Fig. 14.6 *Decompensation of chronic AS with a marginal BP treated with an inoconstrictor.* These PVLs illustrate the impact of the inoconstrictor NE in the decompensated state of AS described in Fig. 14.5. LV Ees has increased; however, the increase in SVR has increased the arterial load to a greater extent. As a result, the EF and SV (~15%) have decreased further. Due to the increase in ESV and SBV (NE-induced venoconstriction), the EDP has increased by ~10%

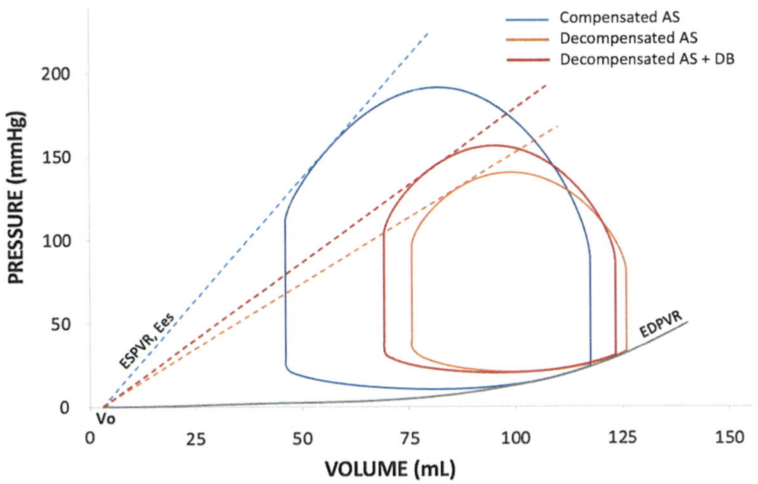

Fig. 14.7 *Decompensation of chronic AS with a marginal BP treated with an inodilator.* These PVLs illustrate the impact of the inodilator DB in the decompensated state of AS described in Fig. 14.5. In this instance, DB was titrated to increase LV Ees to a similar degree as occurred with NE. The increase in LV contractility and modest decrease in SVR and the arterial load increase the EF and SV. The BP has increased due to a greater increase in CO than decrease in SVR (98/82 to 105/88 mmHg). A decrease in ESV and SBV (DB-induced venodilation) has decreased the EDP by ~10%
Comparing the inodilator to inoconstrictor, the SV is ~20% greater with the inodilator; thus, so too are the mean and peak transvalvar pressure gradients (~20%). As a result of the differing effects of the two agents on the arterial resistance vessels and venous capacitance vessels, the EDP is also significantly lower with the inodilator

References

1. Stout KK, Verrier ED. Acute valvular regurgitation. Circulation. 2009;119:3232–41.
2. Carabello BA. Aortic stenosis. N Engl J Med. 2002;346:677–82.
3. Bernard S, Deferm S, Bertrand PB. Acute valvular emergencies. Eur Heart J Acute Cardiovasc Care. 2022;11:653–65.
4. Carabello BA, Crawford FA Jr. Valvular heart disease. N Engl J Med. 1997;337:32–41.
5. Peterson KL. Severe calcific aortic stenosis. J Am Coll Cardiol. 2005;46:299–301.
6. Saikrishnan N, Kumar G, Sawaya FJ, et al. Accurate assessment of aortic stenosis: a review of diagnostic modalities and hemodynamics. Circulation. 2014;129:244–53.
7. Ternacle J, Clavel MA. Assessment of aortic stenosis severity. Cardiol Clin. 2020;38:13–22.
8. Zaid RR, Barker CM, Little SH, et al. Pre- and post-operative diastolic dysfunction in patients with valvular heart disease. J Am Coll Cardiol. 2013;62:1922–30.
9. Briand M, Dumesnil JG, Kadem L, et al. Reduced systemic arterial compliance impacts significantly on left ventricular afterload and function in aortic stenosis. J Am Coll Cardiol. 2005;46:291–8.
10. Baumgartner H, Hung J, Bermejo J, et al. Recommendations on the echocardiographic assessment of aortic valve stenosis: a focused update from the European association of cardiovascular imaging and the American society of echocardiography. J Am Soc Echocardiogr. 2017;30:372–92.

11. Llyod JW, Nishimura RA, Borlaug BA, et al. Hemodynamic response to nitroprusside in patients with low-gradient severe aortic stenosis and preserved ejection fraction. J Am Coll Cardiol. 2017;70:1339–48.
12. Garcia D, Barenbrug PJC, Pibarot P, et al. A ventricular-vascular coupling model in presence of aortic stenosis. Am J Physiol Heart Circ Physiol. 2005;288:H1874–84.

Chapter 15
Right Ventricular Function and Pulmonary Hypertension

Nirica Borges and Ronald A. Bronicki

Pulmonary hypertension is common to a variety of conditions occurring in patients presenting to an intensive care unit. A fundamental understanding of the right ventricle (RV) and its response to an increase in afterload is essential to the care of critically ill patients. Here, we discuss the anatomy and function of the RV, the determinants of the pulmonary arterial load, and the interaction between the RV and pulmonary arterial system.

The RV and left ventricle (LV) have similar gene expression and protein composition and thus appear to have similar processes of excitation and contraction [1, 2]. There are however significant differences between the two ventricles in terms of their anatomy, the role of ventricular interdependence on ventricular function, and, most importantly, their respective afterloads and in turn muscle mass.

The anatomical arrangement of cardiomyocytes for each ventricle differs considerably [1–2]. LV subepicardial and subendocardial cardiomyocytes are predominantly obliquely oriented, which cause the LV to twist and shorten in a wringing-like action. The RV contains longitudinal subendocardial myocytes that cause longitudinal shortening in a peristalsis-like manner from inlet to outlet, accounting for approximately 75% of RV contraction, and a superficial layer of circumferentially oriented fibers that results in a bellows-like motion of the free wall toward the septum.

The ventricles have an intimate anatomical relationship. Both ventricles are bound together by spiraling muscle bundles, which encircle both ventricles in a complex interlacing fashion. Both atria and ventricles share a common septum, and all chambers are contained within and constrained by the pericardial membrane. This anatomic relationship sets up a continuous physiologic interplay between the two ventricles throughout the cardiac cycle, leading to diastolic and systolic ventricular interdependence [1–4]. These interactions describe how the change in

---

N. Borges · R. A. Bronicki (✉)
Baylor College of Medicine, Texas Children's Hospital, Houston, TX, USA
e-mail: nmborges@texaschildrens.org; rxbronic@texaschildrens.org

R. A. Bronicki et al. (eds.), *Simulation in Cardiovascular Critical Care Medicine*, https://doi.org/10.1007/978-3-031-63557-1_15

volumes and pressures of one ventricle affects the volumes and pressures of the other. Under normal conditions, LV stiffness and diastolic pressure are greater than for the RV, causing septal deviation into the RV during diastole. And because afterload is considerably greater for the LV, septal deviation into the RV continues into systole. If, however, the RV is volume loaded, as seen, for example, with an atrial septal defect, RV diastolic volume and pressure increase. When this occurs, the normal diastolic transeptal pressure gradient is reduced or reversed, in which case the septum assumes a midline position or deviates into the LV, respectively. This diastolic ventricular interaction reduces the effective compliance of the LV. When RV afterload increases, RV volume and pressure are elevated throughout the cardiac cycle, altering the position of the septum during systole as well.

LV contraction contributes to RV pressure generation [3, 4]. Studies have demonstrated double-peaked waveforms for RV pressure during isovolumic contraction, where one waveform results from RV free wall contraction and the other component from LV contraction, the latter mediated by the interventricular septum. The greater the LV systolic pressure and septal deviation into the RV, the greater the developed ventricular pressure. Systolic ventricular interaction contributes to upwards of 40% of RV pressure generation.

Interventricular interdependence plays a central role in the pathophysiology of low cardiac output in pulmonary hypertension-induced RV failure. Decreased RV output coupled with RV distension and adverse diastolic ventricular interaction decreases LV filling and its ability to generate pressure, decreasing LV assistance to RV ejection, precipitating a positive feedback cycle [3–6].

The factor most responsible for the difference between RV and LV function is their respective afterloads and in turn corresponding muscle mass. The determinants of the pulmonary arterial load are the same as for the systemic circulation. However, the magnitude and distribution of the components that comprise the arterial load are quite different.

As with the systemic arterial load, the determinants of pulmonary arterial impedance based on the three-element Windkessel model are characteristic impedance, resistance, and compliance [7–10]. Under normal conditions, resistance is some ten times greater and compliance one-third less for the systemic arterial circulation compared to the pulmonary arterial circulation. In addition, the distribution of compliance is quite different [7–10]. In the systemic circulation, compliance is primarily located in the proximal aorta, while in the pulmonary circulation, it is distributed throughout the circuit. Changes in each component contribute to acute and chronic changes in the arterial load for both circulations [8]. Another important difference between the two circulations is that the pulmonary artery occlusion pressure (PAOP) contributes much more to the pulmonary arterial load than does the central venous pressure (CVP) to the systemic arterial load [11]. This is discussed further below.

The low pulmonary arterial load results in a trapezoidal RV pressure volume loop (PVL). RV output starts early during pressure generation, resulting in brief isovolumic periods. The low arterial load also allows for antegrade flow into the pulmonary artery (PA) to continue despite the onset of RV relaxation. Nearly 60% of RV stroke volume is ejected after peak RV systolic pressure occurs. The interval

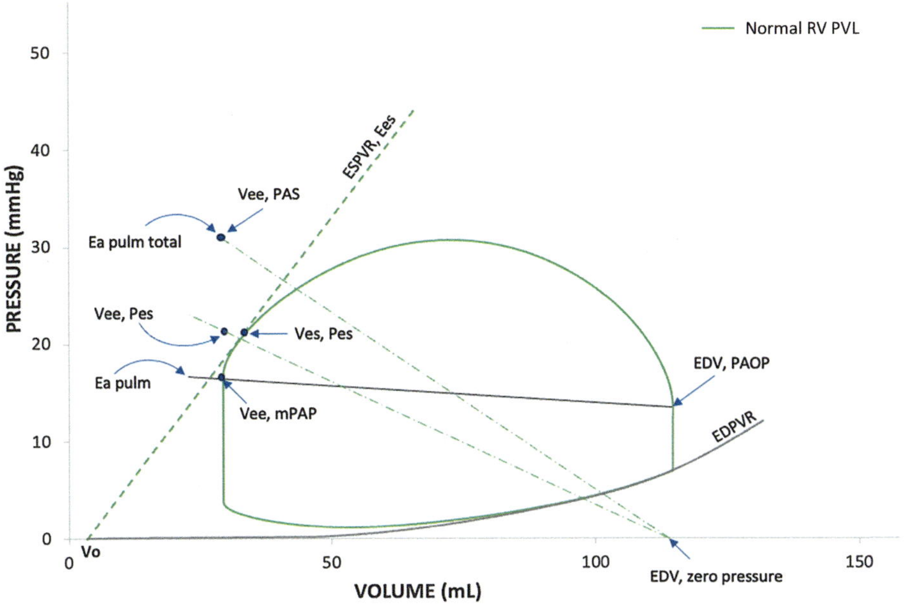

Fig. 15.1 *RV PVL under normal conditions.* As discussed, Ea pulmonary is depicted as the slope between the mean PA pressure (mPAP) and volume at end ejection (Vee) coordinate and the EDV and LV EDP or PAOP coordinate, whereas Ea pulmonary total is depicted as the slope between the PA systolic pressure (PAS) or Pes and Vee coordinate and the EDV at zero pressure coordinate

from the time RV pressure falls below PA pressure to the closure of the pulmonary valve is referred to as the "hangout period" (Fig. 15.1) [1, 2, 5, 6]. As discussed above, the differences in ventricular afterload are responsible for the behavior of the interventricular septum. As a result, the RV appears crescent-shaped and the LV bullet-shaped in cross section throughout the cardiac cycle. With increases in the pulmonary arterial load, the hangout period is truncated, and the PVL of the RV shifts from a trapezoidal shape to a rectangular shape, with well-developed isovolumic and relaxation periods, indistinguishable from a normal LV PVL.

Right Ventricular-Pulmonary Artery Coupling

It has been established that when pulmonary arterial impedance is low, a subpulmonic ventricle is not required to generate adequate cardiac output [5, 6]. This principle is exemplified in the Fontan circulation, where a compensatory increase in the stressed blood volume and in turn mean systemic pressure provides a sufficient upstream pressure to drive pulmonary blood flow (see Chap. 5). In fact, in the setting of isolated RV congestive heart failure (e.g., Ebstein's anomaly) and a normal pulmonary arterial load, cardiac output will increase significantly by excluding the RV and adverse diastolic ventricular interaction [12–14].

The same concept of systemic ventricular arterial coupling that was discussed in the chapter on elastance (Chap. 2) may be applied to the RV and pulmonary circulation. If the arterial load (Ea) and RV afterload (PA systolic pressure) increases to a greater extent than RV contractility (elastance, Ees), RV-PA uncoupling ensues causing the ejection fraction and stroke volume to decrease. Thus, it is the magnitude and rate of rise in RV afterload and thus the time allotted for compensatory RV concentric hypertrophy that determine the impact of an elevated pulmonary arterial load on RV output.

Take, for example, the infant with a large, nonrestrictive ventricular septal defect and/or aorta to PA communication. At birth the pulmonary arterial load decreases significantly; however, RV pressure and afterload remain systemic. As a result, RV muscle mass increases at the same rate and to the same extent as for the LV [15, 16]. Left unrepaired, Eisenmenger syndrome will likely develop. RV systolic function is maintained well into adult life in the majority [15, 16]. Patients with Eisenmenger syndrome fare far better than patients with all other forms of pulmonary hypertension [15–17]. Morbidity and mortality are more likely related to systemic hypoxemia, polycythemia, and systemic embolization than RV systolic heart failure.

On the other hand, an acute even modest increase in pulmonary arterial load and RV afterload leads to a significant decrease in RV stroke volume. Factors that acutely effect PA impedance include emboli, acidosis and alveolar hypoxia and hypoxic pulmonary vasoconstriction, and the creation of zone I conditions resulting from alveolar overdistension. Accordingly, a compensated RV may decompensate due to an elevation in pulmonary arterial load and RV afterload and/or decrease in contractility.

Applying the Elastance Construct to the Right Heart

As discussed previously in the chapter on elastance, Sunagawa analytically derived algebraic equations to conceive of effective arterial elastance (Ea) as a lumped parameter of the arterial load incorporating both resistive and pulsatile components [18]. This mathematical analysis relies on simplifying assumptions: total peripheral resistance (TPR) = mean arterial pressure (MAP)—CVP / stroke volume (SV) X heart rate (HR). This can be simplified to the following: TPR X HR approximates pressure end systolic (Pes) / SV = Ea [18–23]. The simplifying assumptions are as follows:

1. The CVP is negligible relative to the MAP.
2. The MAP can be approximated by Pes.
3. The end ejection volume (Vee) is equivalent to end systolic volume (Ves).

However, the assumptions required to approximate Ea in the systemic circulation are not valid for the pulmonary circulation.

First, the PAOP is not negligible relative to the mean pulmonary artery pressure even under normal conditions (Fig. 15.1). The PAOP contributes importantly to RV afterload, independent of pulmonary vascular properties. Thus, effective pulmonary arterial elastance, Ea pulmonary total, reflects not only pulmonary vascular properties (Ea pulmonary) but also the influence of downstream pressure (the PAOP). Second, based on the nature of the RV-PA interaction described above, RV ejection continues past the point of end systole. As a result, Vee and pressure end ejection are smaller than Ves and Pes, respectively (Fig. 15.1). However, as discussed, with elevated RV afterload, the hangout period is lost, and the PVL of the RV shifts from a trapezoidal shape to a rectangular shape, with well-developed isovolumic and relaxation periods, indistinguishable from a normal LV PVL. Thus, in the setting of pulmonary hypertension, Ea pulmonary total can be approximated by Pes/SV and depicted as the negative slope connecting the end systolic pressure volume coordinate with EDV at zero pressure coordinate. Ea pulmonary is reflected in the negative slope connecting the EDV and PAOP coordinate with the mean PA pressure and Ves.

Simulations

In the following simulations (Figs. 15.2, 15.3, 15.4, 15.5, 15.6, 15.7, 15.8, 15.9, and 15.10), we illustrate the differences in RV and LV function and loading conditions for a normal circulation; the impact of acute pulmonary hypertension on RV output

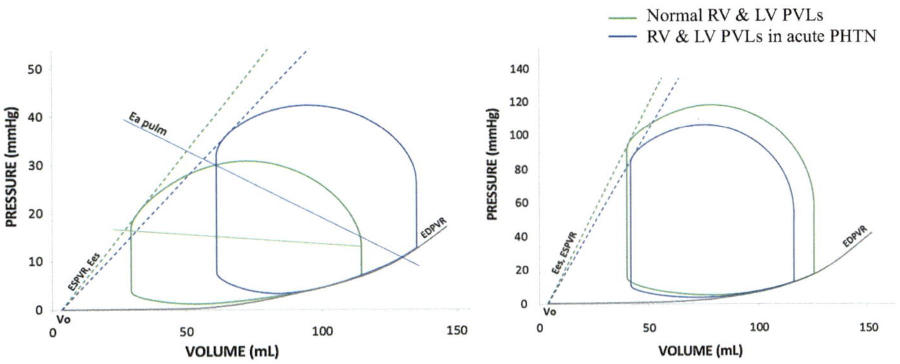

Fig. 15.2 *Acute, moderate PHTN.* These PVLs illustrate the impact of acute PHTN resulting from sepsis induced acute respiratory distress syndrome (ARDS). RV PVLs on the left, LV PVLs on the right. Biventricular systolic function (Ees) is decreased. PVR is elevated, pulmonary arterial compliance is decreased. As a result, Ea pulmonary (depicted), and thus Ea pulmonary total (not depicted), is elevated. As a result of the increase in Ea pulmonary total/Ees, RV EF and SV are decreased, and the ESV elevated (see Chap. 2). The increase in ESV coupled with neurohormonal activation-induced venoconstriction and increase in SBV (see Chap. 5) increase the RV EDV and EDP. Despite the decrease in LV Ees, the LV EDV and EDP are reduced due to the decrease in RV SV. The increase in Ea pulmonary total was greater than the decrease in RV Ees, resulting in the increase in RV Pes as well as mean and systolic PA pressures

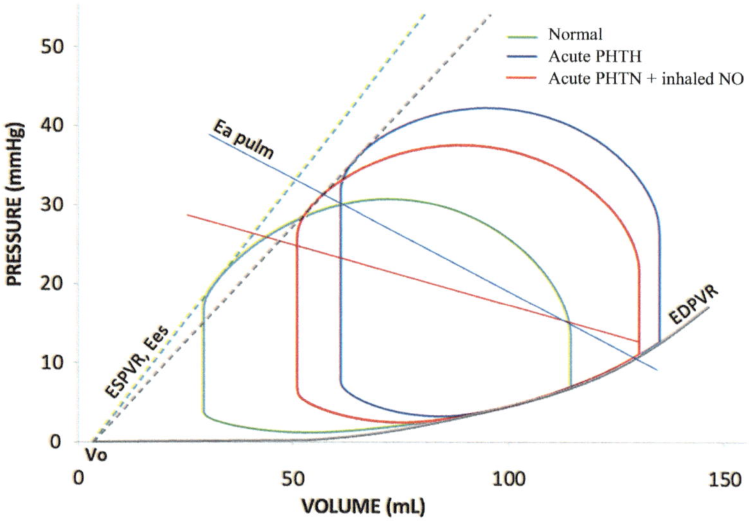

Fig. 15.3 *Acute, moderate PHTN treated with a vasodilator.* These RV PVLs illustrate the impact of the selective pulmonary vasodilator inhaled nitric oxide in the same patient with ARDS-induced pulmonary hypertension discussed in Fig. 15.2. Ea pulmonary is reduced. As a result, Ea pulmonary total/Ees is reduced and thus RV EF and SV increase, the RV ESV decreases. Pes decreases as Ees is unaffected and Ea pulmonary total decreases. The LV EDV (LV PVL not depicted) is restored, and the LV EDP increases

and the effects of therapies; the PVL for an RV that has undergone hypertrophy and restored RV-PA coupling, followed by its uncoupling from the pulmonary circulation; and the impact of left-sided heart disease and pulmonary venous hypertension on RV afterload. Included in the simulations is the development of secondary tricuspid regurgitation (TR). TR is frequently associated with pulmonary hypertension resulting from increased left atrial pressure and/or pulmonary arteriolar disease. Increased RV afterload leads to RV dilation and dysfunction, leaflet tethering, tricuspid annulus dilation, and malcoaptation.

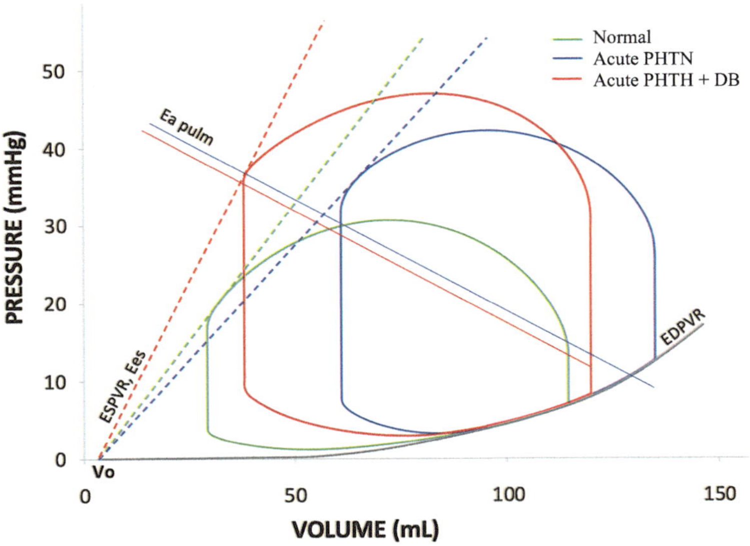

Fig. 15.4 *Acute, moderate PHTN treated with an inodilator.* These RV PVLs simulate the impact of the inodilator DB in the same patient with ARDS-induced PHTN discussed in Figs. 15.2 and 15.3. While DB has modestly decreased PVR, Ea pulmonary remains unchanged (depicted) due to the increase in HR. DB has restored RV contractility. As a result, Ea pulmonary total (not depicted)/ RV Ees decreases, the EF and SV increase, and the ESV decreases. Because RV Ees has increased and Ea pulmonary total is unchanged, Pes as well as mean and systolic PA pressures increases (the PAOP is minimally affected). Thus, despite its vasodilatory properties, DB has increased PA pressures and RV afterload. The decrease in RV ESV coupled with DB-induced venodilation and decrease in SBV have caused the RV EDV and EDP to decrease

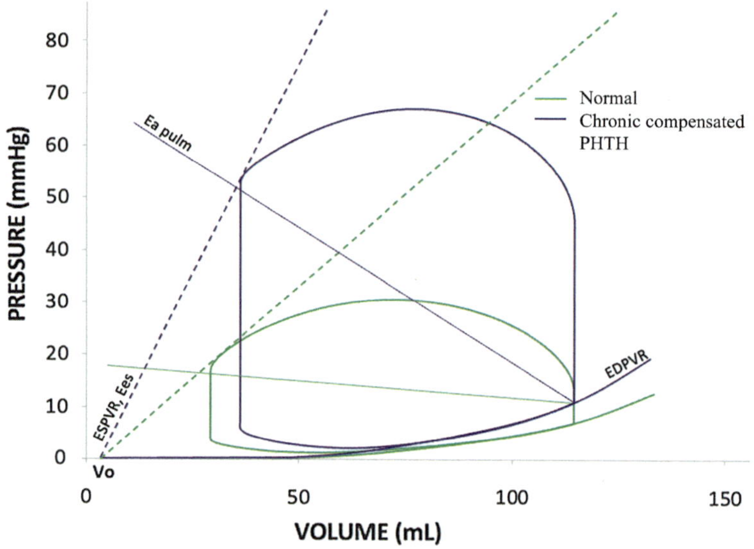

Fig. 15.5 *Chronic compensated PHTN.* These RV PVLs illustrate the differences between a RV with normal function and loading conditions and a RV which has been chronically exposed to elevated RV afterload due to elevated Ea pulmonary and thus Ea pulmonary total (not depicted). Ventricular remodeling has led to concentric hypertrophy and a commensurate increase in RV Ees. Ea pulmonary total/Ees has nearly normalized and thus so too has the RV EF and SV. Of note, despite the significant increase in RV afterload, restoration of RV PA coupling results in a RV EDV that is not elevated. The increase in muscle mass has increased the RV muscle mass/EDV ratio increasing RV stiffness, which is reflected in a shift of the EDPVR up and to the left

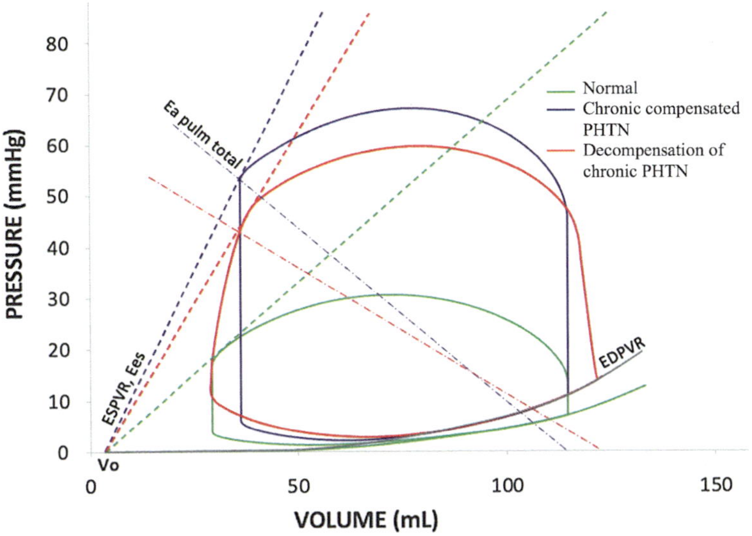

Fig. 15.6 *Decompensation of chronic PHTN.* These RV PVLs illustrate the progression from the chronic compensated state discussed in Fig. 15.5 to a decompensated state. RV contractility has decreased, PVR has increased, and tricuspid regurgitation (TR) has developed

With TR, the isovolumic contraction phase of the cardiac cycle is absent. RV ejection starts with regurgitant flow as soon as ventricular pressure rises above right atrial pressure. The isovolumic relaxation phase of the cardiac cycle is absent as well. Following pulmonary valve closure regurgitation continues as ventricular pressure is greater than right atrial pressure. Regurgitation reduces RV volume until RV pressure falls below right atrial pressure

In this instance, the TR is only moderate in severity (RF of 36%). With TR, the forward or total SV (regurgitant plus forward) may be used to determine Ea pulmonary total. Ea pulmonary total based on the total SV reflects the total afterload on the RV, both the arterial load and low impedance pathway provided by the right atrium. As a result of the TR, Ea pulmonary total has decreased. And because Ea pulmonary total has decreased to a greater extent than Ees, the EF increases appreciably despite the increase in PVR and decrease in RV contractility

The total SV has increased; however, the forward SV has decreased, causing the PA pressure to fall (68/46, mean of 51 to 60/42, mean of 46 mmHg). Despite the increase in PVR, PA pressures and RV afterload have decreased. Of note, additional ventricular remodeling has not occurred as RV Vo is unchanged

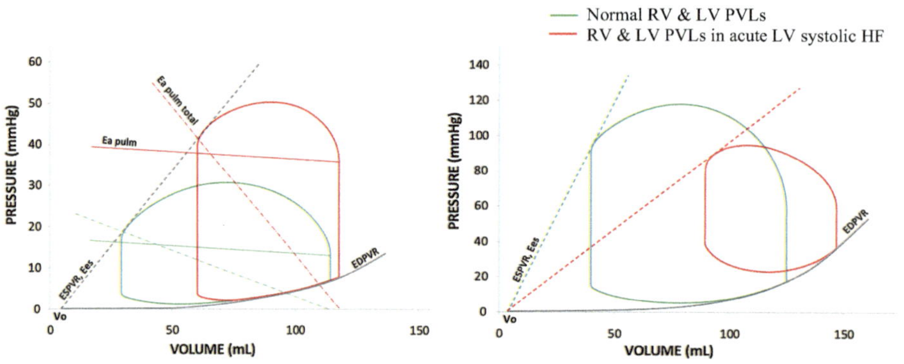

Fig. 15.7 *Acute LV systolic HF induced PHTN.* These PVLs illustrate the impact of an elevated LV EDP on the pulmonary arterial load in acute LV systolic HF. RV PVLs on the left, LV PVLs on the right. In this instance, pulmonary vascular properties (Ea pulmonary) are unaffected. However, Ea pulmonary total is elevated, illustrating that the PAOP contributes importantly to RV afterload independent of vascular properties. Ea pulmonary total/Ees has increased significantly, and thus RV EF and SV have decreased significantly

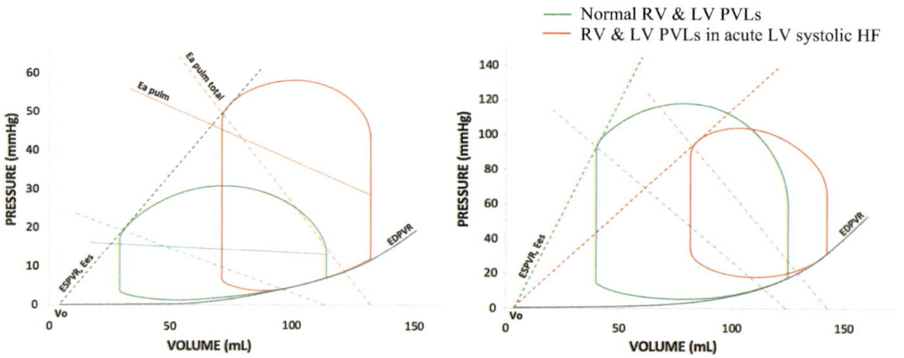

Fig. 15.8 *Acute LV systolic HF induced PHTN.* RV PVLs on the left, LV PVLs on the right. These PVLs illustrate that increase in PA pressure and RV afterload is due to an increase in Ea pulmonary total, resulting from alterations in pulmonary vascular properties (increase in PVR, decrease in compliance) and increase in Ea pulmonary, as well as an increase in LV EDP and PAOP. RV Ees is unchanged. Thus, the increase in Ea pulmonary total/Ees causes the RV EF and SV to decrease. The increase in RV ESV coupled with a decrease in venous capacitance and increase in SBV, increase the RV EDV and EDP

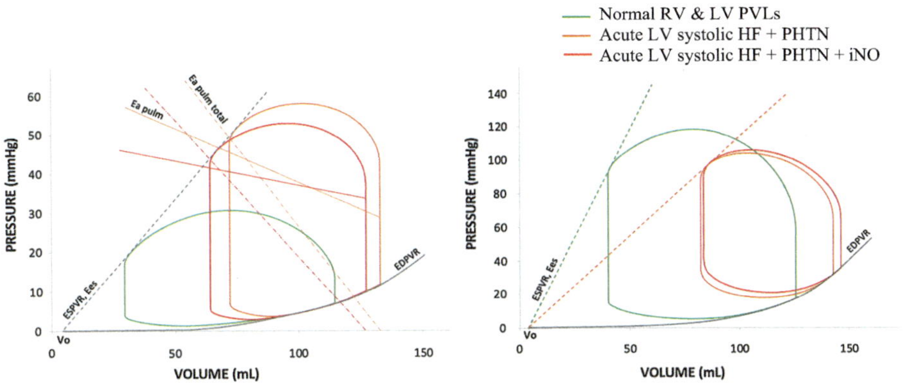

Fig. 15.9 *Acute LV systolic HF induced PHTN treated with inhaled nitric oxide (iNO).* These PVLs illustrate the impact of iNO on biventricular loading conditions in the same patient discussed in Fig. 15.8. RV PVLs on the left, LV PVLs on the right. Inhaled NO selectively vasodilates the pulmonary circulation. In this instance, iNO has decreased PVR from 4.7 to 1.8 WU and Ea pulmonary decreases significantly. However, the increase in RV SV increases the LV EDV and EDP (+6 mmHg), which partially offsets the iNO-induced decrease in Ea pulmonary. As a result, the decrease in Ea pulmonary total and Ea pulmonary total/RV Ees is limited, and thus so too is the increase in RV EF and SV

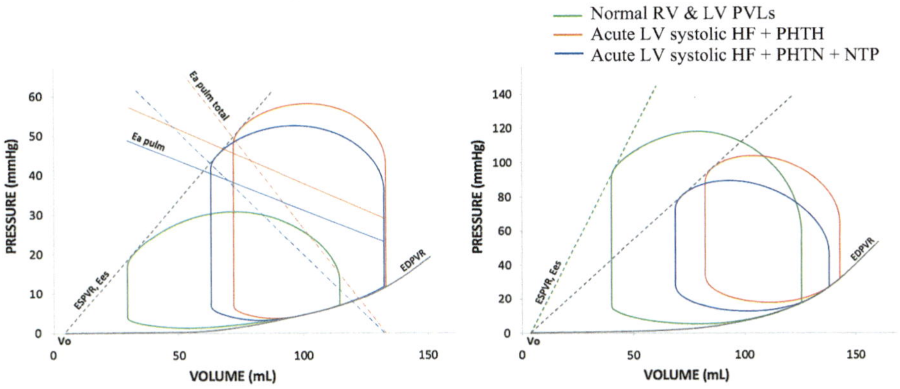

Fig. 15.10 *Acute LV systolic HF induced PHTN treated with NTP.* These PVLs illustrate the impact of vasodilator NTP in the same patient discussed in Figs. 15.8 and 15.9. RV PVLs on the left, LV PVLs on the right. NTP vasodilates venous capacitance as well as systemic and pulmonary arterial resistance vessels. In this instance, low dose NTP was used. It was titrated to maintain the minimum accepted mean and systolic systemic arterial pressures. Ea systemic is reduced, decreasing LV ESV. This coupled with vasodilation of venous capacitance vessels and a decrease in SBV, decrease the LV EDV and EDP. The decrease in Ea pulmonary and PAOP decreases Ea pulmonary total. As a result, Ea pulmonary total/RV Ees decreases, the EF and SV increase. Concurrently, Ea systemic/LV Ees has decreased, increasing LV EF and SV significantly. The net effect is an increase in SV and CO and decrease in LV EDP by ~15% for each parameter

References

1. Penny DJ, Redington AN. Function of the left and right ventricles and their interactions between them. Pediatr Crit Care Med. 2016;17:S112–8.
2. Friedberg MK, Redington AN. Right versus left ventricular failure. Differences, similarities, and interactions. Circulation. 2014;129:1033–44.
3. Dell'Italia LJ. The right ventricle: anatomy, physiology, and clinical importance. Curr Probl Cardiol. 1991;16:659–720.
4. Dell'Italia LJ. Anatomy and physiology of the right ventricle. Cardiol Clin. 2012;30:167–87.
5. Sanz J, Sanchez-Quintana D, Bossone E, et al. Anatomy, function, and dysfunction of the right ventricle. J Am Coll Cardiol. 2019;73:1463–82.
6. Konstam MA, Kiernan MS, Bernstein D, et al. AHA scientific statement. Evaluation and management of right-sided heart failure. Circulation. 2018;137:e578–3622.
7. Noordegraaf AV, Westerhof BR, Westerhof N. The relationship between the right ventricle and its load in pulmonary hypertension. J Am Coll Cardiol. 2017;69:236–43.
8. Chemla D, Lau EMT, Papelier Y, et al. Pulmonary vascular resistance and compliance relationship in pulmonary hypertension. Eur Respir J. 2015;46:1178–89.
9. Saouti N, Westerhof N, Postmus PE, et al. The arterial load in pulmonary hypertension. Eur Respir Rev. 2010;19:197–203.
10. Thenappan T, Prins KW, Pritzker MR, et al. The critical role of pulmonary arterial compliance in pulmonary hypertension. Ann Am Thorac Soc. 2016;13:276–84.
11. Tedford RJ, Hassoun PM, Mathai SC, et al. Pulmonary capillary wedge pressure augments right ventricular pulsatile loading. Circulation. 2012;125:289–97.
12. Takagaki M, Ishinno K, Kawada M, et al. Total right ventricular exclusion improves left ventricular function in patients with end-stage congestive right ventricular failure. Circulation. 2003;108:II-226–9.
13. Goldstein JA, Barzilai B, Rosamond TL, et al. Determinants of hemodynamic compromise with severe right ventricular infarction. Circulation. 1990;82:359–68.
14. Goldstein JA, Vlahakes GJ, Verrier ED, et al. The role of right ventricular systolic dysfunction and elevated intrapericardial pressure in the genesis of low output in experimental right ventricular infarction. Circulation. 1982;65:513–22.
15. Hopkins WE. The remarkable right ventricle of patients with Eisenmenger syndrome. Coron Artery Dis. 2005;16:19–25.
16. Hopkins WE, Waggoner AD. Severe pulmonary hypertension without right ventricular failure: the unique hearts of patients with Eisenmenger syndrome. Am J Cardiol. 2002;89:34–8.
17. Daliento L, Somerville J, Presbitero P, et al. Eisenmenger syndrome. Factors relating to deterioration and death. Eur Heart J. 1998;19:1845–55.
18. Sunagawa K, Maughan WL, Burkhoff D, et al. Left ventricular interaction with arterial load studied in isolated canine ventricle. Am J Phys. 1983;245:H773–80.
19. Kelly RP, Ting C-T, Yang T-M, et al. Effective arterial elastance as index of arterial vascular load in humans. Circulation. 1992;86:513–21.
20. Brener MI, Burkhoff D, Sunagawa K. Effective arterial elastance in the pulmonary arterial circulation. Circ Heart Fail. 2020;13:e006591.
21. Brener MI, Masoumi A, Ng VG, et al. Invasive right ventricular pressure-volume analysis: basic principles, clinical applications, and practical recommendations. Circ Heart Fail. 2022;15:e009101.
22. Brener MI, Burkhoff D, Sunagawa K. Response by Brener et al to letter regarding article "effective arterial elastance in the pulmonary arterial circulation: derivation, assumptions, and clinical applications". Circ Heart Fail. 2020;13:e0071117.
23. Tedford RJ, Hsu S, Kass DA. Letter by Tedford et al regarding article, "effective arterial elastance in the pulmonary arterial circulation deviations, assumptions, and clinical applications". Circ Heart Fail. 2020;13(5):007081.

Index

R. A. Bronicki et al. (eds.), *Simulation in Cardiovascular Critical Care Medicine*, https://doi.org/10.1007/978-3-031-63557-1

GPSR Compliance

The European Union's (EU) General Product Safety Regulation (GPSR) is a set of rules that requires consumer products to be safe and our obligations to ensure this.

If you have any concerns about our products, you can contact us on ProductSafety@springernature.com

In case Publisher is established outside the EU, the EU authorized representative is:

Springer Nature Customer Service Center GmbH
Europaplatz 3
69115 Heidelberg, Germany

Batch number: 10158117

Printed by Printforce, the Netherlands